Quadruple T

CW00927336

Obesity, Sleep Apnea, Diabetes, and Heart Disease

By Delilah Banks

Timely Publishing

Why you need to read this book

Before we begin, can you do me a favor? The next time you're walking down the streets of your city or town, take a look around you. How many people are obviously, uncontrollably, morbidly obese? And next time you're in casual conversation with a friend...why don't you discuss how many of your other friends and loved ones are battling heart disease (and how many have passed away?)

Next...

Do some research as to how many young children are diagnosed with diabetes before they've even had the chance to experience life.

The truth is this:

There is something seriously wrong with our modern society! We are getting sicker and weaker by the day, and it's mostly because of our disastrous lifestyle choices. I'm talking about things like junk food, which contains high levels of fat, sugar, and salt...smoking, drugs, and alcohol...sedentary lifestyles spent in front of the computer or T.V....and constant stress and worry. All of which lead to deadly health conditions.

This book focuses on just four on these conditions.

I call them the "quadruple threat," and they include obesity, sleep apnea, diabetes, and the big one—heart disease. This is not a random grouping. I've chosen to do this because all four of these diseases are in some way intertwined, and exacerbate each other. (They're like an evil Fantastic Four, in a way.) These are truly the four great plagues of our era. And in this book I will go over every one in great detail.

You'll learn how and why they develop...what you can do about them...plus little-known facts and tips for easing your suffering. Make no mistake—these conditions are deadly. If you've suffered through the agony of losing a loved one to something like a heart attack, you already know this.

But there is hope.

This book is going to go a long way towards educating you about these ailments and helping you to potentially avoid them.

Table of Contents

Why you need to read this book
Part One – Obesity
An Introduction to Obesity
Obesity: An Overview
The Role of Genetics
The Role of Behavior
Are All Calories Created Equal?
Food Addiction
Is This My Fault?
Lifestyle Changes
Treatment Options: Pharmaceutical and Surgical
Behavioral Modification: Mindset and Expectations
Obesity Wrap-up
Part Two – Sleep Apnea
An Introduction to Sleep Apnea
The Value of Sleep
What Is Sleep Apnea?
Who Is at Risk?
Obesity and Sleep Apnea
Symptoms of Sleep Apnea
The Dangers of Sleep Apnea
Diagnosing and Treating Sleep Apnea
Breathing Devices for Sleep Apnea
Oral Appliances for Sleep Apnea
Surgeries for Sleep Apnea
Alternative Treatments and Home Remedies
Sleep Apnea Wrap-up
Part Three – Diabetes
An Introduction to Diabetes
What Is Diabetes?
How Diabetes Affects Your Body and Health, Directly and Indirectly
Diabetes Demographics
Maintaining a Healthy Weight: Fat, Protein, and Carbohydrates Explained
Lifestyle Changes to Undo Diabetes
How to Stay Motivated and Track Your Progress
Medications
Diabetes Wrap-up
Part Four – Heart Disease

An Introduction to Heart Disease
What Is Heart Disease?
Signs, Symptoms, and Risk Factors
The Connection with Diabetes
Warning Signs (Stroke and Heart Attack)
What to Do About It
Where Should I Start?
Steps to Reducing High Blood Pressure and Unclogging Your Arteries
Superfoods—Eat Your Way to a Healthy Heart
Reversing Heart Disease for Life
Alternative Treatments for Heart Disease
Heart Disease Wrap-up
Copyright

An Introduction to Obesity

Obesity is a complex issue that stems from biological, environmental, and cultural factors. This book takes you through the ins and outs of how to identify obesity, how to understand where it comes from, and how to make adjustments to enjoy your lifestyle. Weight management is a very personal choice—whether you are underweight or obese—and it helps to understand the factors at play.

<u>Obesity: An Overview</u>

Adiposity is defined as the state of being "fat" or obese. The benchmarks for the terms "overweight" and "obese" are defined by the body mass index (BMI) measurement. Adults can calculate their BMI by measuring their height and squaring that number. Then, divide your weight in pounds by your height in inches squared. Then multiply that number by 703. The result is your BMI. Here is an example:

Alice is 5'9" (69 inches). She weighs 180 pounds. Her calculation would go like this:

$180/(69*69) = 180/4761 = .037807$
$.037807*703 = 26.6$
Her BMI is 26.6

Males and females do their calculations the same way.

John is 5'8" and weighs 210 pounds. His BMI is calculated as follows:

$210/(68*68)=.045415$
$.045415*703=31.9$
His BMI is 31.9

A BMI below 18.5 is considered underweight, and a BMI between 18.5–24.9 is considered healthy weight. A BMI between 25–29.9 is overweight, and a BMI above 30 is obese (CDC: Defining Overweight and Obesity). So, Alice is just barely above the overweight marker and John is considered to be obese.

This method of calculation has a few drawbacks. Some individuals weigh more because they have higher muscle concentration. Therefore, their BMI is larger but it doesn't accurately reflect their body fat concentration. BMI is widely accepted as accurate, though, for the average person.

So, why does a person become obese? What makes people so different that some can be on the extremely underweight side of the spectrum and some can be on the extremely obese side of the spectrum? Some want to blame genetics, while some want to solely blame environment. The truth is probably closer to a combination of the two—a "multifactor explanation."

The Role of Genetics

Genetics play an important part in how your body stores fats and converts dietary fats to energy. They can even determine if you have a propensity to overeat or be overly sedentary. Your genes are the instructions your body has to respond to its changing environment, and they are unique to only you. People from the same ethnic and racial background—and the same family—share key parts of their genes.

While direct, conclusive evidence tying genes to obesity is still being sought after, indirect evidence among families, sets of twins, and adopted children strongly suggest that genetics significantly influence obesity. Scientists cannot pinpoint a specific gene that causes one to be overweight. They don't even have a solid idea of which groups of genes could be factors. But through studies it is widely believed that genes work in complicated ways with environmental and behavioral factors to influence some people towards obesity (CDC: Public Health Genomics).

Genetics testing for obesity is only in its early stages. In the coming years, scientists and doctors will have a clearer idea of how genetics affects weight gain. Until then, doctors do know to screen patients for potential influencing factors, such as having a family member who has heart disease or type II diabetes. While someone cannot change their family history, doctors encourage people that are at higher risk for health problems to adjust their behaviors and environment to promote healthy practices.

The Role of Behavior

Behavior plays just as important a role in obesity as genetics does. The average weight of developed or developing countries has greatly increased over the last several decades, and this increase can be attributed to a variety of interconnected behaviors (Cancer Research UK: The Causes of Obesity).

1. Fast food has created a convenient, unhealthy alternative to natural food. Many people are turning to fast food because it is quicker and cheaper than cooking for themselves or buying healthy foods. Fast food is processed and rich in calories, fat, carbohydrates, sugar, and sodium. All of those pre-packaged ingredients work together to create an unhealthy combination.

2. Not only are fatty foods more available, but the food industry has learned how to make their products taste better and last longer. This all happens through the use of additives and preservatives, neither of which are natural or good for the body.

3. There is a widespread acceptance of soft drinks. These are calorie- and sugar-rich drinks that are often offered in serving sizes that vastly outweigh the body's ability to process them. Along with that, there are other drinks like beer, juice from concentrate, energy drinks, enhanced coffees, and others that are dripping with sugar. For an interesting look at the worst drinks, visit http://organic.wonderhowto.com/inspiration/20-worst-drinks-america-0116436/.

4. Sedentary lifestyles are the final behavioral factor that plays into obesity. We now have a lot more jobs that require a person to sit behind a desk instead of getting outside and performing manual labor. On top of that, the widespread use of cars instead of walking or cycling has increased the time that we are not engaging in activity. Along those lines, watching TV and playing on the computer have become more popular pastimes, neither of which expend physical energy.

All of these factors combine to encourage a culture of obesity. On another level, their widespread acceptance has "weeded out" some peoples' genes that encourage healthy eating. For example, the "thrifty genome theory" says that our ancestors had genes that would allow them to sustain themselves through long periods of drought or food scarcity. Over time, those genes were either lost or suppressed, due to how easily accessible food is today. The less active that people are and the more unhealthy their appetite is, the more likely they are to lean towards obesity.

Weight gain can be avoided, though, so we have to ask: Why does it happen? The ill effects of being obese are well documented in certain cancers, heart disease, diabetes, joint pain, etc. So why do people "let" themselves become obese? Is that even an accurate description of the problem? We know that obesity stems from genetics and behavioral factors, but what else is at play here?

Are All Calories Created Equal?

Scientists and doctors have made great strides in defining and treating obesity. The way that obesity has evolved into an epidemic is a fairly new phenomenon, so there is still more progress to be made in this field of study. Like all scientific discoveries, first a hypothesis is made. Then, if it proves true, it is widely held as a workable theory. The thing is, new discoveries or breakthroughs can debunk well-known theories.

Consider when Galileo challenged the scientific and religious community with his radical idea that the universe did not in fact revolve around the Earth. Scientist of that day were correct in saying that there was a sun, and that the pieces (planets, even though they didn't fully understand them) of the universe moved. But they were incorrect as to how they moved. Nutritionists have had similar changes in their theories over time.

The laws of thermodynamics play an interesting role in health culture. The first and second laws are as follows:

1. First law of thermodynamics: Heat is a form of energy. Because energy is conserved, the internal energy of a system changes as heat flows in or out of it. Equivalently, perpetual motion machines of the first kind are impossible.

2. Second law of thermodynamics: The entropy of any isolated system never decreases. Such systems spontaneously evolve towards thermodynamic equilibrium—the state of maximum entropy of the system. Equivalently, perpetual motion machines of the second kind are impossible.

The first law is important because calories are a measure of heat, or energy. This intuitively makes sense because we eat to sustain ourselves with energy. For a long time it was widely believed that "a calorie is a calorie," regardless of what food the calorie is made up of. This works with the second law, because it implies that all things are equal, or are working to be equal.

In practice, this would mean that 100 calories of pasta (high in carbohydrates) would cause the same weight gain as 100 calories of eggs (low in carbohydrates). Without several key studies done in the last 10 years or so, "a calorie is a calorie" would still be the prevailing theory.

In fact, Authoritynutrition.com has compiled the findings and synopses of 23 key studies that explain how not all calories are created equal. If all calories are not equal, which ones are the best to consume? These studies show that a diet low in carbs (versus low in fats) may be the best way to lose weight.

Below are a few trials that have debunked the theory that the best way to lose weight is to control fat intake. Each uses a randomized pool of subjects (the best way to conduct accurate experiments) and is published in well-respected journals.

1. Foster GD trial of a low-carb diet for obesity, published in the *New England Journal of Medicine* 2003

This trial took 63 obese individuals and randomly divided them into a low carb (LC) group and a low fat (LF) group. The LF group was calorie restricted but the LC group was not. The groups were dieted for 12 months.

While both groups lost weight (so both methods are effective), the LC group lost 7.3% of their body fat, while the LF group only lost 4.5% of their body fat. That's a significant difference! The results stayed significantly different for the first 6 months, but by the 12-month point the LC group reverted to only losing about 6.5%.

Weight loss wasn't the only thing measured. The LC group had greater improvements in blood triglycerides and HDL (the "good" cholesterol), but other factors like insulin sensitivity and fasting blood glucose were statistically the same.

2. Samaha FF trial of a low-carb diet for severe obesity, published in the *New England Journal of Medicine* 2003

In this trial, 132 severely obese individual (average BMI of 43) were divided randomly into an LC and an LF group. Just as above, the LF dieters were calorie restricted. Many of these participants suffered from obesity-related diseases such as metabolic syndrome and type II diabetes. The study went on for six months.

As in the last study, the LC group lost more weight. This time, the LF group lost an average of 4.2 pounds while the LC group lost 12.8 pounds—three times as much! Other factors also leaned in favor of the LC group. Triglycerides and fasting blood glucose went down by 38 mg and 26 mg respectively in the LC group, and only by 7 mg and 5 mg in the LF group. Insulin levels went down in the LC group by 27%, but slightly increased in the LF group. Also, insulin sensitivity improved in the LC group, but slightly increased in the LF group.

3. Sondike SB trial of a low-carb diet for overweight adolescents, *The Journal of Pediatrics* 2003

This trial studied 30 overweight adolescents divided into an LC and an LF group for 12 weeks. Neither group had to restrict their calories. The study found that the LC group lost 21.8 pounds and the LF group lost 9 pounds, a significant difference. The LC group also had significant decreases in triglycerides and non-HDL (the "bad") cholesterol.

These trials work together to prove that not all calories are equal. Perhaps more important than counting calorie intake is to consider the make-up of those calories. For a while it was thought that if you restricted your fat intake, you would lose fat. These studies show that restricting your diet, whether it is on a fat basis or a carb basis, is an effective way of losing weight. These carb-based studies, though, prove that if you actually focus on restricting your carbohydrates, and focus more on eating natural fat- and protein rich-foods, you will lose more weight. You will also enjoy the benefits of other health increases more than you would on a restricted fat diet.

Food Addiction

Food addiction greatly parallels any other kind of addiction, including drug addiction. When some people eat certain highly palatable foods, defined as foods rich in sugar, sodium, and fat, their brains release the feel-good drug dopamine. Dopamine can actually be released in a variety of ways. Exercise releases dopamine, which is often explained as the "runner's high" that can cause people to go as far as an unhealthy addiction to running that eventually tears down their joints and overworks their hearts.

The release of dopamine in a food addiction situation convinces the eater that they need to keep eating, even though they are not hungry. Consider how many salty potato chips you can eat in one sitting. Even when you've passed the point of full, you want to eat more because of how "satisfying" the feeling is. That is the work of dopamine convincing you that you need more.

Food addiction can also lead to a food tolerance. People who are addicted to food can start out with moderate portions, but every time they eat they feel like they need more food to be satisfied. This could be a result of the dopamine, or the unhealthy foods could actually be desensitizing them to how much they've consumed.

Food addicts, just like drug addicts, will continue to abuse themselves, despite negative consequences like unwanted weight gain, emotional trauma related to the weight gain, social stigma, or relationships damaged by the addiction. They may try to stop their addiction by themselves, but it often proves to be very difficult and frustrating.

Not everyone who suffers from food addiction is obese, or even overweight. Like it was pointed out in the genetics section, some people have genes that better help them convert extra calories into energy, instead of storing it as body fat. Some people compensate by exercising, even though they still suffer from the addiction.

Having a food addiction can be a very personal matter that should be approached with sensitivity—but it can be helped. Below are some questions to ask yourself (or consider in another person's situation) to decide if you are suffering from addiction:

- Did I plan to eat that much of _____? (Fill in whatever fatty, salty, or sugary food you are drawn to.) Consider how much you thought you were going to eat when you started. Did you eat significantly more?
- Am I having a hard time justifying how much I ate, or did I not realize how much I was eating?
- Did I keep eating, even when I wasn't hungry anymore?
- Did my overeating cause me to feel sick, but I kept going?
- How far would I be willing to go to obtain certain unhealthy foods? Is that abnormal?
- Am I so interested in eating certain foods that I would sacrifice time that I could be working, spending time with family, or participating in hobbies, religious activities, or family traditions? How much do I value these foods? Do I consider them more important than the other parts of my life?
- Does the fear of overindulging keep me away from certain people, places, or activities where certain fatty foods will be present? How much do I stress myself about steering clear of these things?
- Does my desire for certain foods keep me from effectively performing on the job, in school, or as a member of society?

These are all questions that you have to answer for yourself. If you said yes to more than one of them, you should consider the possibility that you have a food addiction.

The problem with addictions is that society tells people to "fix themselves" or "get some self-control," while neither of those may be the real solution. People who suffer from addiction often try to fix the problem themselves, but go through setbacks that derail their efforts. Consequently, they will often console themselves for their failures through the thing that brings them peace: the dopamine rush that comes from food. It is easy to see how this can turn into a vicious cycle.

The negative effects of food addiction can be seen through:

- Physical withdrawal symptoms. When you cut back on certain foods, do you go through anxiety, agitation, or other abnormal physical changes?
- Eating certain foods sends you through cycles of pleasure coupled with depression, guilt, or self-hate. Really consider how eating (or not eating) certain foods makes you feel.

- You increasingly want to eat more of the unhealthy foods to combat negative emotions. These emotions can stem from the stigma of addiction, weight gain, failed dieting attempts, strained relationships, or frustrating encounters with family and friends who are genuinely concerned but ultimately unhelpful (authoritynutrition.com).

Addiction is an ugly, horrifying reality. Consider the other addictions that you know. Why do smokers, alcoholics, and drug abusers keep doing what they do? It's not because they want to kill themselves. It's because they are addicted to that substance.

Nobody wants to be fat, overweight, or obese. Nobody wants to suffer from diabetes, a failing heart, arthritis, or joint pain. Yet they keep eating the foods that cause their problems. It's simply because they are addicted to that food.

Addiction isn't something you just get over, either. It usually tears your life apart, ruining relationships and job opportunities before a person is brought so low that they break the addiction on their own. Consider an alcoholic that loses his job and his family because of his addiction. Through rehab, intense self-control, and community support, he can lay down the bottle and move on with his life. But just one drink—just a single drink—can bring his addiction back in full force. The same is true for food addicts. You can beat your addiction, but just one taste of the harmful food you used to love can send you right back to where you were. It's horrible, but it is the truth of addiction (authoritynutrition.com).

The important thing to remember is that there are now trained professionals who can help and motivate you. Your friends and family may not be the most helpful at first, even though they are desperately trying to assist you. Remember that their not understanding where you are coming from is more our society's lack of understanding and less them actively trying to offend you.

<u>Is This My Fault?</u>

Some 35% of American adults over the age of 20 are obese—and 69% of Americans over 20 years old are overweight. Even 12% of children as young as 2–5 years old are obese, and 18% of children between the ages 5–19 are obese (CDC: Obesity and Overweight).

A logical connection can be made between the fact that if you are overweight as a child, you are more likely to be overweight or obese as an adult. Do children really have control over whether they are obese? Probably not. The responsibility probably lies somewhere between American food culture, unhealthy ingredients, the abundance of cheap unhealthy food, sedentary lifestyles, the higher costs of healthier foods, misinformation, weight gain-inducing conditions, and personal choice. No single one of these factors can be singled out as the sole perpetrator, so it isn't fair to berate yourself with questions about whether this is your fault.

More important is to understand your condition and what you can do to live a healthy lifestyle. The first step is to understand why you are here—wherever that is for you. You may be borderline overweight; you may be obese. Consider what got you here. Was it unhealthy, fast food choices? Was it a medical condition you had no control over? Was it a hormone imbalance? Was it a controllable lack of physical activity?

Now figure out how you feel about it. Is your weight threatening your health, or does it not affect you enough for you to want to change? Weight loss is a personal, complex choice. You have the options of modified diet and exercise, which may not interest you. You have the options of weight loss pills or surgery, but they can have negative side effects and complications. Consider whether or not you want to lose weight, and how far you want to go.

Now you have to understand that other people may not agree with or understand your choices—but they are still yours to make. To quote msnbc.com contributor Joan Raymond from her article "Heavy Burden: Fat but not My Fault" concerning American's bias against overweight people:

> Because obesity and all of its co-morbidities like heart disease, stroke, diabetes, some cancers, and asthma, to name a few, rack up big health care bills (according to a 2009 CDC study, America now spends as much as $147 billion annually on the direct and indirect costs of obesity)

some researchers fear this bias might get worse as health care reform plays out.

"There is some evidence that shows that for whatever reason weight bias is increasing," says obesity researcher Robert Carels of Bowling Green University in Ohio. His own research published in the journal Eating and Weight Disorders shows a "strong level of contempt" for the obese, especially among people who believe the weight is highly controllable. "There's a feeling of why should I have to pay for them (the obese), if they can do something about their weight," says Carels. "As a society we have a strong, pull-yourself-up-by-the-bootstrap mentality, and the overweight are the targets."

If you are overweight, you have probably suffered from bias or backlash. The important thing to remember is that there are people out there in the same boat as you, trying to find the same solutions you are looking for. You can reach out and be a part of a supportive community. There are steps you can take to control your weight, ranging from daily activities to medical procedures.

<u>Lifestyle Changes</u>

It is well known that weight is gained by consuming more calories than you burn. This goes back to the First Law of Thermodynamics. The law says that energy (in our case, calories) cannot be destroyed, just shifted around. So, you can only lose weight by using up the calories you consume.

We use calories in different ways. Just going about your day and walking across the house or your office burns a certain number of calories without you having to think about it. Your metabolism also burns calories without you having anything to do with it. Like we said in the genetics section, everyone's metabolisms work differently. Exercise is the most direct way to burn calories because you have control over how hard you are working.

The simple explanation about calories consumed minus calories burned is a little misleading. For that to be the whole truth, plain and simple, it would have to be true that all calories are equal. Since we have proven that all calories are not equal, it is fair to look at the effects of calories from different foods. Different calories do affect your hormones and metabolism in different ways.

The two foods we are going to consider are soda and eggs. Soda is an unhealthy drink, in part because it is sweetened with high-fructose corn syrup (HFCS), which is even worse for you than regular sugar. Both sugar and HFCS are made up of two simple sugars—glucose and fructose. Glucose is naturally present in a lot of foods, including starches like potatoes. Your body produces glucose on its own, and all cells have glucose in them, so it is an unavoidable part of our diet (Healthy Eating).

Fructose is much different, though. Until recently, it was never a major part of humans' diets (except in ripe fruit). The only organ in your body that can break down fructose is the liver. When the fructose is dumped into your liver, it tries to convert it into glucose and store it as glycogen. If your liver is too full of glycogen, though, the fructose will be turned into fat. That fat will then be moved around the body or left to clog up the liver. This leads to weight gain, liver failure, and all the other health issues associated with those problems.

Eggs, on the other hand, are a major source of protein, and the body breaks them down in a very different way. About 30% of protein calories are burned during their digestion. The protein is then used to suppress appetite and increase your metabolism. Protein also aides in the creation and restoration of muscles, which are metabolic tissues that naturally burn calories on their own. Compared to soda, it is very easy to see that the effects of calories via sugar versus the effects of calories via protein are very different (Authority Nutrition).

So now that we understand the importance of a good diet, what role does exercise play in losing weight? First, losing weight is not the only objective to obtain before having a healthy lifestyle. That's why we need to couple a balanced diet with exercise—to reap the health benefits of both. There are articles, like the one put out by *Time* in 2009 titled "Why Exercise Won't Make You Thin," that claim that exercise is a trivial part of losing weight. The article leads readers to believe that exercise can be counterproductive to living a healthy life. That seems to defy everything we've ever been taught about health, right?

Well, the article makes a very good point that is worth considering. Exercise is the one direct way to burn calories, and burning calories is a way to lose weight. (Remember the basic formula that calories consumed minus calories burned equals weight gain? If the "calories burned" half of the equation is greater than calories consumed, you will lose weight.) The article points out that while exercising burns calories, it also stimulates hunger. So if someone who does an intense workout and burns 500 calories goes out and eats fast food right after to reward themselves, they haven't been productive at all. They might as well not have worked out and just skipped the fattening food.

Nothing about that assertion is incorrect. Exercise could lead to weight gain if someone isn't conscious about how they are conducting themselves. An intense workout doesn't justify consuming a large amount of calories. But here are some big points that the article misses or doesn't explain fully:

- Losing weight without exercise is certainly possible, but it isn't easy. Some people are physically incapable of exercising, and some people hate to exercise, but they still lose weight. The problem, though, is that a healthy lifestyle isn't all about weight loss. There are several other benefits of exercise.
- Exercise boosts your metabolism—especially lifting weights. Anything you do to build muscle will increase your metabolism and burn calories long after you stop working out, because muscles are metabolic tissues that work around the clock. Exercise also uses up excess calories that the body might otherwise store as fat.

- Exercise releases that feel-good drug called dopamine, which has a myriad of positive effects on the body. It keeps you feeling good long after your workout, it gives you a boost of self-esteem, it lowers your stress levels, and it helps you sleep better at night.
- Moderate aerobic exercise may actually curb hunger. This was reported by *Today Health* after the release of two articles by the journal *Metabolism* and Brigham Young University. Weight lifting was not found to have the same effect, though.
- Exercising creates an atmosphere of healthiness. While this may not be true for everyone, it certainly is a general rule. When someone goes through the hard work of exercising, they aren't going to want to blow their progress on a few unhealthy snacks. It can also eliminate emotional eating that is tied to dissatisfaction over weight loss not achieved by dieting alone.

Exercise and a healthy diet are great ways to manage weight. But in extreme cases there may be other avenues available that are worth considering.

<u>Treatment Options: Pharmaceutical and Surgical</u>

Weight loss drugs, part of the pharmaceutical efforts to lower weight, are recommended for use in extreme cases. For instance, someone who is overweight should first try diet and exercise to bring themselves back down into the healthy BMI category. If that isn't working or they become obese, there are over-the-counter, herbal, and prescription drugs available. When consulting a doctor, weight loss drugs are usually prescribed to those with a BMI>30 (obese), and a BMI>27 (overweight) if there are risk factors for weight-related diseases like type II diabetes, heart disease, hypertension, etc.

There are a variety of drugs available in both approved and unapproved tiers, so one should do their research and work closely with a medical professional before committing to any. The first tier of drugs are the non-FDA approved dietary supplements or herbal remedies, the most common of which are Hydroxycut and Trimspa. These remedies usually have caffeine and an herb that suppresses appetite, and they are available over the counter. Because of the caffeine used, these drugs can increase heart rate, cause insomnia or tremors, increase acne, or incite restlessness (lifescience).

Trimspa includes the ingredient glucosamine. This ingredient extends the amount of time that glucose stays in the bloodstream after a meal, which causes the user to feel full longer. It does have the potential, though, to induce an insulin resistance, which could lead to type II diabetes.

There is another over-the-counter drug called Alli (main ingredient: orlistat) that is not FDA approved, but blocks fat absorption in the intestine. As explained above, excess sugar is converted by the liver into fat and either stored there or sent to other parts of the body. Alli blocks that fat from being absorbed in the liver and causes about 30% of the fat to be excreted as waste. Users may notice oily spotting, urgent bowel movements, oily stools, or flatulence, especially if they are eating a diet high in fat. It is important to note that Alli also prevents nutrient absorption (lifescience).

The second tier of weight loss drugs are the prescription FDA-approved diet pills. These are often appetite suppressants, or "anorectics." The most common include:

1. Adipex-P, which has the active ingredient phentermine and helps to suppress appetite
2. Belviq, which has the active ingredient lorcaserin and helps to promote a feeling of fullness (selective serotonin 2C receptor agonist)
3. Bontril PDM and Bontril SR, which have the active ingredient phendimetrazine and help to suppress appetite
4. Desoxyn, which has the active ingredient methamphetamine and helps to suppress appetite (can be very addictive and cause reliance and abuse, and lead to illegal distribution)
5. Didrex, which has the active ingredient benzphetamine and helps to suppress appetite
6. Diethylpropion, which has the active ingredient diethylpropion and helps to suppress appetite
7. Qsymia, which has the active ingredients phentermine and topiramate (extended-release capsules help to suppress appetite; the effect of topiramate on weight loss is unknown)
8. Suprenza, which has the active ingredient phentermine and helps to suppress appetite

(Information provided by Drugs.com)

As you can see, all of these affect the appetite or feelings of fullness to try and curb the perceived need to eat. They all come with their own risks that a health professional can help you assess.

It is generally safe to lose one to two pounds per week. Weight loss drugs can only help someone lose between 5–10% of their weight over a year, when coupled with reasonable diet and exercise (drugs.com). Here's an example:

Mike is 5'8" and weighs 210 pounds. His BMI is calculated as follows:

$210/(68*68)=.045415$
$.045415*703=31.9$
His BMI is 31.9, so he is obese

If Mike lost the max safe amount of weight through diet and exercise, he would lose two pounds per week, meaning more than 100 pounds a year. With Mike's height, it would not be healthy for him to lose that much weight. Instead, he should shoot for a BMI between 18–24.5. That would mean his weight range would be:

BMI 18 for 68" = X pounds
18/703=.025604
.025604*(68*68)= 118 pounds
BMI 18 for 68" = 118 pounds

BMI 24.5 for 68" = X pounds
24.5/703=.034851
.034851*(68*68)= 161 pounds
BMI 24.5 for 68" = 161 pounds

To have a healthy BMI, Mike only needs to lose 50 pounds. Over 52 weeks, he could lose a little less than one pound per week and be in the healthy BMI range a year from now.

With dietary pills, he would lose 5–10% of his weight in the next year.

210 – 5%(210) = 199.5 pounds
210 – 10%(210) = 189 pounds

Although he can't lose weight as fast, dietary pills could get him 21 pounds closer to his goal in just a year. The next year he could lose another 5–10%.

Year 2: 199.5 - 5%(199.5) = 189.5
189 - 10%(189) = 170.1

Year 3: 189.5 - 5%(189.5) = 180.0
170.1 - 10%(170.1) = 153.1

In just three years, Mike could lose more than the weight he needs to have a healthy BMI using diet pills and a reasonable lifestyle. Prescription and over-the-counter weight loss drugs are usually prescribed as a second attempt effort at losing weight when the patient is incapable of exercising. Any lifestyle can be improved with diet management and exercise, which are both highly recommended.

One of the main issues with any of these diet pills, whether they are over-the-counter or prescription drugs, is that appetite suppressants can trick your body into going into "starvation mode." If you aren't eating enough calories to sustain you, your body will slow down its metabolism and hoard calories. You will start storing all the fat that you can, because your body is uncertain when it will need those calories. This is the body's natural defense mechanism against starvation, and it can cause you to gain significant weight. The best advice is to consult with your doctor or nutritionist on what is a safe diet for your, and which diet pills, if any, are best for you to take.

Remember that since obesity is a relatively new issue, the science behind its cures is still being developed. What is claimed today as a revolutionary diet pill could come out years from now as having serious health implications that doctors simply don't understand right now. There are always unknowns as to how a diet pill suppresses appetite and how that affects normal food breakdown (livescience). People who should not take weight loss drugs are those who have diseases or disorders that can be exasperated by the drug, as well as pregnant women. Always consult with your doctor before starting weight loss pills, because doctors are equipped to help you understand the associated side effects and risks.

In even more extreme cases, surgical measures may be necessary to lose weight. This should be reserved as an option that is considered after regular diet and exercise have failed. These procedures come in two kinds: restrictive and malabsorptive/restrictive surgeries. Solely malabsorptive surgeries (intestinal bypasses) are no longer available because the risks involved were too extreme compared to the benefits.

Restrictive surgeries work to shrink the size of the stomach, which slows down digestion. The stomach can be shrunk from its normal size of about three pints down to one to three ounces. This drastically reduces the amount of food that can be eaten in one sitting. Since the digestion is moving slower, you also feel full for longer. These are the less invasive of the two options, and the surgeries can usually be reversed.

1. Adjustable gastric banding is a restrictive type of surgery. Doctors will take an inflatable tube and wrap it around the stomach to divide it into two connecting sections. The upper section will be smaller and initially hold the consumed food. As food is being digested, it will slowly move through the opening to the larger, lower section of the stomach. Patients can typically eat one half to one cup of well-chewed or soft food in a sitting.

This surgery is one of the least invasive options possible, with only a small incision and special tools. There is less risk of complications than with a more invasive surgery, and your recovery will go faster. Once the band is in place, it can be loosened or tightened by a doctor removing or adding more saline solution. The band can also be removed. The weight loss is going to be conservative, though, and patients may be more at risk to regain the weight over several years.

Side effects include vomiting from eating too much, since your stomach isn't used to being restricted. The band can also create it's own complications by slipping, loosening by itself, and leaking. These issues will require more surgeries, but they are not typically life threatening (WebMD).

2. A sleeve gastrectomy is a slightly more invasive surgery that is irreversible. It could be the first step in a series of surgeries that become more invasive, should a patient continue to need to lose weight.

In this surgery, about 75% of the stomach is removed, leaving someone with only the max capacity to consume about ¾ pint. This surgery is the safest step towards weight loss when a patient is considering a gastric bypass or a biliopancreatic diversion. Both of these procedures could be done a year or so after the sleeve gastrectomy if they are needed.

Obese patients who have a sleeve gastrectomy usually lose more than 50% of their excess weight, but since the procedure is relatively new, the long-term effects have not been observed yet. Like all surgeries, there are risks of complications and infections, and the sleeve has the potential to leak. The surgery could also cause blood clotting (WebMD).

Malabsorptive/restrictive surgeries change how you digest food in addition to restricting your stomach. These procedures make it harder for your body to absorb calories by removing or bypassing part of the digestive tract. Their main complication is that while you aren't absorbing as much fat, you also will be missing out on key nutrients, and will have to eat an adjusted diet for the rest of your life. These surgeries are invasive, and cannot be reversed except for in extreme cases.

1. Gastric bypasses are one of the most common types of weight loss surgeries. Doctors will go to the stomach (either through minimally invasive or open surgeries) and divide it into an upper and lower section. The upper section, which would first hold the consumed food, is directly connected to the small intestine. This greatly restricts the surface area for calories to be absorbed into the body.

Gastric bypasses can have amazing, dramatic effects. Patients usually lose 50% of their desired weight in the first six months, and can keep losing weight for the next two years. Weight-related problems like diabetes, arthritis, high cholesterol, and lack of sleep tend to clear up very quickly. A dramatic improvement to quality of life can be achieved in a short amount of time, and the results usually last for 10 years or more. Gastric bypass does come with its own drawbacks, though.

This type of surgery complicates the body's ability to absorb nutrients. You can suffer serious medical issues if you don't take dietary supplements accordingly. You will have to continue to take the supplements for the rest of your life. Another complication is that you can suffer from "dumping syndrome." This is where food is moved too quickly from the stomach to the intestines, and it causes you to be sick and bloated, and suffer pain, sweating, and diarrhea. These effects are most commonly triggered by foods high in carbohydrates and sugar, which causes some professionals to consider "dumping syndrome" a positive side effect, because it encourages you to stay away from those unhealthy foods.

A patient risks having complications and infections with the surgery. The mortality rate of these surgeries is only 1%, but that is higher than purely restrictive procedures. The rapid weight loss can put you at risk for forming gallstones, and patients risk developing hernias long after having the surgery (WebMD).

2. A more intense version of gastric bypass is the biliopancreatic diversion. This procedure eliminates up to 70% of the stomach. The remaining portion is connected to a lower part of the small intestine. This procedure can give you even greater weight loss than the gastric bypass. For the long term, 70–80% of excess weight is kept off. You are also left with more stomach than a gastric bypass or a gastric banding, so you can eat more at one time without feeling nauseous.

Biliopancreatic diversions are still less common than bypasses, or are at least the second part of a sequence of procedures, because you are more likely to suffer from nutritional deficiency. Dumping is also still a possibility. You suffer the same risk of hernia and gallstone as with a bypass, but the mortality rate is higher, between 2.5–5%. This method should only be used in extreme cases when there aren't other weight loss options and the weight is detrimental to the patient's health (WebMD).

As always, consult with your doctor on what surgery is the best fit for you. Weight loss surgeries are typically recommended in the following cases:

1. You are severely obese (BMI>40).
2. You are obese (BMI 30–35) but also have weight related issues like diabetes, heart disease, high cholesterol, etc.

3. You have tried and failed to lose weight in other ways. Surgery can be complicated and should be used as the last resort.

Unless you have already had a weight loss surgery, doctors will probably try to start you out with the least invasive option possible (WebMD). While all doctors should be licensed professionals, it never hurts to get several professional opinions and consider your payment options.

What are some other ways that you can control your quality of life? Typically, weight goals will not be achieved overnight, and setbacks or slow results can become discouraging. In the next section we will talk about realistic expectations.

<u>Behavioral Modification: Mindset and Expectations</u>

Now that we have talked about the causes of obesity, day-by-day steps to curb weight gain, and your medical options, we are going to delve into what you should expect from yourself. When you are trying to lose weight, here are a few tips to keep you motivated and happy with your changing lifestyle:

1. First, congratulations on your decision! You want a healthier lifestyle, and that's great. It takes a lot for someone to admit that they aren't happy with themselves enough to want to change.

2. Don't forget that lasting change doesn't usually happen overnight. A new lifestyle requires commitment and perseverance.

3. Don't be discouraged when you don't lose weight like you expected to. We see ads on TV or hear about amazing transformation stories. If that's you, that's great! But if it isn't, it's easy to be left discouraged. Like we've said, everyone has different genes that control their bodies differently. Some people may lose a lot of weight in the first weeks of their program, while others are several weeks in and barely seeing progress. That's okay. As long as you are working with a proven system (I'd suggest talking to your doctor or nutritionist) you know you're on the right track.

4. Make sure you are working with a proven system! There is nothing more frustrating than working hard towards something that is counterproductive.

5. A safe amount of weight to lose is between 0.5–2 pounds per week. Crash diets can ruin your metabolism and cause you to gain back all the weight you lost and more.

6. Finally, weight loss ebbs and flows. Just during the day, your weight can fluctuate back and forth. Different times of the month can cause you to gain weight, like when a woman is going through PMS.

When you want to lose weight, your overall goal should be set for the long term and you should be flexible with your expectations when you first start out. It may take a little trial and error to decide what works best for you, but the important thing is that you are on the right path.

<u>Obesity Wrap-up</u>

Now that you know where you stand, what should you do about it? You have a lot of options!

If you feel that you simply need a lifestyle modification, consider the information in the Role of Behavior and Diet/Exercise sections. First, just becoming more active will go a long way to reducing your weight and making you feel better. But never forget the important role that a healthy diet plays. Below are two examples of a beginner low-carb diet and a beginner workout schedule.

Don't eat: sugar (soft drinks, fruit juices, agave, candy, ice cream and many others); highly processed foods (if it looks like it was made in a factory, don't eat it); "diet" and "low-fat" products (many dairy products, cereals, crackers, etc.); artificial sweeteners (aspartame, saccharin, sucralose, cyclamates, and cesulfame potassium—use Stevia instead); high omega-6 seed and vegetable oils (cottonseed, soybean, sunflower, grapeseed, corn, safflower, and canola oils); trans fats ("hydrogenated" or "partially hydrogenated" oils); gluten grains (wheat, spelt, barley and rye—includes breads and pastas).

Eat: meat (beef, lamb, pork, chicken, and others—grass-fed is best); fish (salmon, trout, haddock, and many others—wild-caught fish is best); eggs (omega-3 enriched or pastured eggs are best); vegetables (spinach, broccoli, cauliflower, carrots, and many others); fruits (apples, oranges, pears, blueberries, strawberries); nuts and seeds (almonds, walnuts, sunflower seeds, etc.); high-fat dairy (cheese, butter, heavy cream, yogurt); fats and oils (coconut oil, butter, lard, olive oil, and cod fish liver oil). Drink water, coffee, and tea. In moderation, eat tubers (potatoes, sweet potatoes), non-gluten grains (rice, oats, quinoa), extremely dark chocolate, and dry wines.

(Information taken from Don't Eat and Eat from http://authoritynutrition.com/low-carb-diet-meal-plan-and-menu/.)

For specific meal ideas, visit http://authoritynutrition.com/low-carb-diet-meal-plan-and- menu/. Remember to consult your doctor or nutritionist before making any more changes to your diet. They should be a helpful resource when deciding what works best for your needs.

Below is a one-week workout schedule for beginners. It includes two days of strength training, because muscles are metabolic tissues that burn calories around the clock. Building muscle is a very effective way to burn calories.

Day 1 Aerobics: 20-minute brisk walk, get your heart rate up

Day 2 Strength Training:

Warm up with stretches for 5–10 minutes

Upper body: 1–2 sets of 8–16 repetitions of 3 exercises using resistance bands or dumbbells.

Lower body: 1–2 sets of 8–16 repetitions for 3 of these exercises: squats, lunges, side step lunges, reverse lunges, calf lifts.

10 minutes of core exercises like planks, twists, lemon squeezes, side crunches.

Day 3 Rest! You can do light aerobic exercise or stretches if you want to, but it's important to give your body a day to recover.

Day 4 Aerobics: 20-minute brisk walk OR walk for 15 minutes and climb up and down the stairs for 5 minutes.

Day 5 Strength Training:

Warm up with stretches for 5–10 minutes

Upper body: 1–2 sets of 8–16 repetitions of 3 exercises using resistance bands or dumbbells (work different muscles than on day 2).

Lower body: 1–2 sets of 8–16 repetitions for 3 of these exercises: squats, lunges, side step lunges, reverse lunges, calf lifts (different exercises than day 2).

10 minutes of core exercises like planks, twists, lemon squeezes, side crunches (different exercises than day 2).

Day 6 Rest! You can do light aerobic exercise or stretches if you want to, but it's important to give your body a day to recover. Prepare yourself for next week!

Day 7 Rest! This is a beginner workout schedule. It's important to set short-term goals for your improvement and not push yourself too hard too fast. Always warm up and cool down before and after working out. Remember to keep yourself limber by stretching—it also prevents injuries. Congrats! You made it through the first week.

Workout Information (Day 1 to 7) taken from:
http://www.exercise4weightloss.com/weight-loss-workout.html#Beginner

There are so many variations that can be made to this workout schedule. For more options, look online. The same applies to the low-carb diet plan. You can find full menus that take you through each day with meals and snacks. Get started towards a healthier lifestyle today!

If you think that you or a loved one suffers from food addiction, read back through the signs we pointed out in the Food Addiction section. Proven, positive results have come out of seeing a doctor to treat your addiction. You may be put in therapy sessions with a counselor, given medication, or introduced to a support group. You just have to find something that works for you.

If you want to consider medical means to reduce your weight, make sure that you know the options and risks associated. Start talking with a doctor today. They are the trained professionals who can walk you through the ins and outs of each procedure. Together you can decide what is best for your lifestyle.

Now you have the tools to decide where you want to go from here. Weight management is a very personal choice, and hopefully this text has empowered you to make decisions that are in your best interests.

An Introduction to Sleep Apnea

Apnea (spelled aponea in the United Kingdom and other countries) comes from the Greek word that means to "want for breath." Apnea today is defined as a pause in breathing. When used in the term "sleep apnea," it means a chronic cycle of breathing pauses that happen when one is sleeping. It is a very serious disorder that sometimes goes unrecognized or undiagnosed because its symptoms can be hard to pinpoint. This book will take you through an in-depth study of the underlying causes behind sleep apnea, how it can affect your life, who is most at risk, and what you can do to combat its effects.

The Value of Sleep

Sleep is vital to maintaining health, although it is something that scientist do not fully understand. Scientists and doctors do know, however, that a lack of sleep can cause a variety of health problems.

Your biological clock, also known as your circadian rhythm, is regulated by the changing of dark to light. We become sleepy at night because the lack of daylight produces melatonin, a chemical in our brains that makes us feel tired. During the day, sunlight blocks the production of melatonin so that we can stay awake. This rhythm can be thrown off balance by traveling across time zones, changing work shifts, or excessive use of artificial light (like that of computer and phone screens). It can take several days or weeks after a big change for your clock to reset itself to the schedule that you need.

An important part of keeping your biological clock on track is getting the right amount of sleep. But what is a healthy amount of sleep? That question can be answered differently for different people. The older we get, the less sleep we typically need. As listed on helpguide.org, it is recommended that a newborn up to the age of 2 months requires 12–18 hours; from 3 months to 1 year, 14–15 hours; from 1 year to 3 years, 12–14 hours; from 3 years to 5 years, 11–13 hours; from 5 years to 12 years, 10–11 hours; from 12 years to 18 years, 8.5–10 hours; and from 18+ years, 7.5–9 hours of sleep per night. (Information taken from www.healthguide.org/life/sleeping.htm.)

Your body goes through four different recurring stages while you sleep. These are broken into either REM or non-REM sleep. The stages form a cycle that repeats itself on average every 90 minutes.

The first stage is non-REM stage one, where you are starting to fall asleep. This is when you first go to bed, after you are done thinking about the day, and your mind and body begin to relax. In this stage your muscles are beginning to relax, your eyes might be slowly moving under your eyelids, and you are easily awakened. It lasts about five minutes. Then you enter into non-REM stage two. In this stage your muscles are already relaxed, so your heart rate slows down, your eye movements stop, and your body temperature decreases. This stage can last anywhere from 5-25 minutes. It is the first stage of actual sleep (hclpguide.org).

Next comes non-REM stage three, otherwise known as deep sleep. This is where the body regenerates itself physically. Your body stops emitting alpha and beta brainwaves, and instead switches to the slower theta and delta waves (Depression and Bipolar Support Alliance). You are much harder to wake up, and if you are woken up you will be disoriented and groggy. It may take several minutes for you to be fully awake.

This stage is extremely important for internal maintenance. Your body is totally relaxed, so blood is drawn away from the brain to service your various muscles to rejuvenate them. Deep sleep is where you repair and improve your immune system, stimulate growth and development, and repair your muscle tissue and other parts of your body.

The fourth stage is REM sleep, where most of your dreams happen. This is also an extremely important stage. In REM sleep your heart rate quickens, blood pressure increases, your breathing becomes more shallow, and your eyes move rapidly. This sleep is so important because it is the time when the body rejuvenates the mind (just like deep sleep rejuvenates the body). Here you process information that you have gathered during the day, and you store it as memories. REM sleep is vital for the production of the feel-good chemicals serotonin and dopamine, which will boost your mood once you wake up. It will also restock your supply of neurotransmitters and form neural connections that work to strengthen and improve your memory (helpguide.org).

<u>What Is Sleep Apnea?</u>

Sleep apnea is a chronic condition that causes pauses or breaks in a person's breathing while they are asleep. Once you are asleep, the muscles in the back of your throat relax, more than the average person. Normally, these muscles would provide support to your uvula, soft palate, tonsils, tongue, and the soft walls of your throat. When the support is removed, the parts of your airway close on themselves, causing you to not be able to inhale adequate breath.

The pauses in breath can last up to a minute at a time (though they are usually only 10–20 seconds), and you can have up to 30 breaks in an hour. Overall, this leads to very poor sleep because the pauses in breathing will jolt you awake with a gasping, choking, or snorting sound. Your body senses that you are not getting enough oxygen, so it wakes you up so that you will open your airway. This is the body's natural defense against suffocating (Mayo Clinic).

Since you are not getting sufficient amounts of deep sleep, sleep apnea can lead to daytime exhaustion and irregular sleeping patterns. It can also negatively impact sleeping partners, since they will probably wake up from your snoring or gasping. All of the negative side effects of sleep apnea relating to lack of sleep can also be transferred to affected sleep partners.

Sleep apnea is hard to diagnose because it is not easily observable during a normal doctor's visit, and it is not a disease that would show up in blood tests. It is even hard for people to know that they have sleep apnea themselves. This is because the condition only happens at night, and people often forget that they were continually waking up. Someone living or sleeping with you might be the first to notice your symptoms.

There are two kinds of sleep apnea—obstructive and central—and obstructive is the most common. If one person suffers from both disorders, the combination of the two is entitled "complex sleep apnea."

Obstructive sleep apnea happens when your airway is blocked or collapses during sleep. This blockage is what causes labored, shallow breathing and breaks in breathing. Shallow breathing can lead to very loud snoring as your lungs try to draw in and exhale breath.

Central sleep apnea is a disorder that causes the area of the brain responsible for the breathing function to stop working. With this kind of apnea, you simply stop breathing for a short amount of time because your muscles are not getting the right signals. Since this is a sender/receptor problem, it usually does not induce snoring. This can make it much harder for the patient or a partner to notice the condition. This is less common than obstructive sleep apnea, and is more common in people with certain existing medical conditions (like heart attacks or strokes), those who live at high altitudes, or those who use certain medicines.

Normal Sleep, Snoring, and Sleep Apnea

Healthy adult sleep moves in cycles, as described above, over a 7.5- to 9-hour series. Each cycle is on average 90 minutes, so you should have 5 to 6 cycles per night. You start out in non-REM stage one while your body begins to slow down and relax. You move into stage two after about 5 minutes up until about 25 minutes. After 25 minutes, you are in stage three—deep sleep—for about 45 minutes.

Then you rise up into REM sleep, where your mind is alert and dreaming, but your body is still asleep. This stage brings you to the full 90 minutes, when you will then sink back down into non-REM stage one and start the cycle all over again. Occasionally you will be brought out of sleep due to changing light, noises, the need to urinate, partners snoring, or snoring yourself—and that is normal. You will shift once or twice per hour, possibly without even waking up, to readjust your blood flow.

Light or infrequent snoring is normal and not a sign of sleep apnea. Snoring by itself is caused by vibrations of the parts of your respiratory system (the uvula, soft palate, tonsils, and soft walls of your throat). It can be caused by your uvula or tongue falling over the opening to your throat, or anything else that obstructs the airway (Huffingtonpost). When you assume another position, the snoring should stop. Snoring can also be caused by poor muscle strength in the tongue and throat, an enlarged uvula or soft palate, and bulky throat tissue or enlarged tonsils.

Sleep apnea is a more chronic condition that can be detected by excessive or loud snoring. It is important to know the difference. Things to ask yourself are, how many nights a week do I snore? How loud is my snoring? Do I have other symptoms that would indicate sleep apnea?

<u>Who Is at Risk?</u>

Anyone can have either kind of sleep apnea, from the young to the elderly. But there are different risk factors for the two kinds of sleep apnea that can put you at a greater risk of developing it, as described below.

Factors for disruptive sleep apnea include:

- Carrying excess weight can put you at greater risk because you store fat around your neck. This fat build-up can obstruct your breathing as your tonsils, tongue, and neck walls are weighed down and close over your throat.
- Alcohol or drugs that are considered "downers" relax your muscles, including the muscles in your neck, which can collapse just as if they were being weighed down.
- Smoking increases inflammation and the fluid held in your upper airways, both of which can block natural breathing. Smokers are three times as likely to develop sleep apnea as non-smokers (Mayo Clinic).
- People with larger neck circumferences, whether it be from a naturally stocky build or weightlifting, can have smaller airways, which block easier than regular airways. Males with a neck circumference of 17 inches or greater and females with a neck circumference of 16 inches or greater are at greater risk (Health Central).
- Enlarged tonsils or adenoids and a large overbite can block the airways. This is particularly possible in children.
- Other uncontrollable factors can negatively impact you. African Americans under the age of 35, the elderly over the age of 60, people with a family history of sleep apnea, and those who are born with naturally smaller airways are more likely to develop obstructive sleep apnea (Mayo Clinic).

Factors for central sleep apnea include:

- Heart disorders such as atrial fibrillation and congestive heart failure can cause and be worsened by central sleep apnea.
- Other health issues, like stroke or brain tumors, can impair the brain's ability to transmit signals to the muscles in the throat that control breathing.

- As with disruptive sleep apnea, men and persons older than 60 are at heightened risk (Mayo Clinic).

Below is a breakdown of some sleep apnea statistics:

- Eighteen million Americans have been diagnosed with sleep apnea, which is 6.62% of the total American population.
- In a limited study conducted by the University of California San Diego, 17% of African Americans had sleep apnea, while only 8% of Caucasians had it.
- Between 4 and 9% of American middle-aged adults have sleep apnea.
- Round 10% of American adults over the age of 65 have sleep apnea.
- Between 25 and 40% of people with sleep apnea also have a family member who has sleep apnea.
- Men are twice times as likely to have sleep apnea as women.
- Women are more likely to develop sleep apnea while they are pregnant or after they go through menopause.
- It is estimated that 2 to 4% of Americans have undiagnosed sleep apnea.
- Those with sleep apnea are six times more likely to die in a car accident. The National Highway Traffic Safety Administrations reported that sleepy driving causes 100,000 vehicular accidents, 40,000 injuries, and 1,550 deaths every year.

Untreated sleep apnea can mean you are four times more likely to have a stroke than someone without sleep apnea. Also, you are three times as likely to develop heart disease than someone without sleep apnea. Half of the people with sleep apnea are at risk for hypertension, caused by overworking the heart. (Statistics courtesy of Web MD and the Sleep Disorders Guide.)

It is important to know that not everyone with obstructive sleep apnea snores, and not everyone who snores has sleep apnea. Snoring and things like daytime drowsiness or moodiness can be indicators of sleep apnea. To know for sure, and to receive proper treatment, you should consult your doctor about any problems you are having. If they are not qualified to diagnose a sleep disorder, ask for references to other physicians who have experience in this area.

Obesity and Sleep Apnea

Lack of sleep is directly related to weight gain, but obesity can also be a cause of obstructive sleep apnea. Obesity and sleep apnea have a complicated relationship in which one can cause the other, and the other can worsen the first. The two work together in a complex web that can become a vicious cycle.

First, we will consider how sleep apnea can lead to obesity. When you do not get the recommended amounts of sleep, your body cannot accurately regulate the amounts of the hormone ghrelin that are released into your system. Ghrelin is responsible for stimulating appetite. So, lack of sleep can directly affect the hormone that makes you feel hungry, which prompts you to eat, even when your body does not need the food. Inadequate sleep also decreases the levels of the hormone leptin, which is responsible for indicating that you are full. So, poor sleep like that caused by sleep apnea can mess up the natural balance of ghrelin and leptin, encouraging you to eat when you do not need to and keeping you from knowing that you are full, leading to weight gain.

The disruptive sleep that comes from sleep apnea can lead to daytime sleepiness and exhaustion. This keeps us from being as productive during the day as we would have been, and it discourages us from participating in physically strenuous activities, like exercise. So, if someone has sleep apnea, the lack of good sleep can cause them to put on weight. Then, as they gain more weight, the exhaustion that comes from sleep apnea can discourage them from exercising to lose or maintain weight. And, to top it off, being overweight or obese can worsen sleep apnea.

In 1999 a study was conducted by The University of Chicago to study how sleep affects the body. The study took 11 healthy young adults and restricted their sleep to four hours per night. While the average adult needs seven and a half to nine hours of sleep per night, these participants were racking up a four- to five-hour sleep debt every day. After six days, the young adult's ability to process glucose had declined almost to the levels of a diabetic. Lack of deep sleep creates all kinds of problems for weight gain because it inhibits the metabolism and disrupts normal hormone levels (National Sleep Foundation).

Another study done by The University of Chicago was conducted with healthy men and women who had an average body mass index (BMI). These men and women were divided into two groups. The first group routinely got the recommended seven and a half to nine hours of sleep per night. The second group got less than six and a half hours. Study administrators performed glucose tolerance tests and found that the group who got less sleep was now experiencing hormone fluctuations that could lead to weight gain in the future. That group also had to produce 30% more insulin than the average sleeping group to keep their blood sugar at healthy levels (National Sleep Foundation). This goes to show that losing just one hour of recommended sleep (from seven and a half to six and a half) could have serious consequences.

These studies both show how sleep apnea can lead to weight gain. But obesity is also the number one reason why American adults develop sleep apnea (Web MD). Over half of the people diagnosed with sleep apnea are either overweight or obese (defined as body mass index of 25–29.9 or >30 respectively). For every one point increase in body mass index, there is an associated 14% increase in the risk of developing sleep apnea. A 10% increase in weight results in a six-fold increase in the risk of developing sleep apnea. Therefore, overweight and obese adults are seven times more like to develop sleep apnea than healthy weight adults (Web MD).

Symptoms of Sleep Apnea

Sleep apnea in general can be hard to recognize. Here are some typical symptoms that either you or a sleeping partner can look for:

- Disrupted sleep, stirring every few minutes, waking up frequently
- Loud, disruptive snoring
- Not being able to concentrate during the day
- Irritability or depression that comes from lack of sleep
- Having a sore throat or dry mouth when you wake up
- Headaches in the morning
- Inability to stay awake during the day, inability to sleep at night
- Difficulty remembering things
- Inability to focus or remember things during the day

As explained before, central sleep apnea is harder to notice than obstructive sleep apnea because of the lack of snoring, but the two do share several of the same symptoms. Some symptoms of central sleep apnea to look for include:

- Abnormal sleeping patterns due to abnormal breathing
- Waking up suddenly with shortness of breath
- Abnormal fluctuations in mood, due to stress
- Hypersomnia: excessive sleeping during the day
- Insomnia: the inability to sleep at night
- Headaches in the morning

The Dangers of Sleep Apnea

Leaving sleep apnea untreated can be dangerous and cause much more serious health problems. If you do not seek treatment, your sleeping habits will continually suffer. You will not be able to maintain the necessary levels of deep sleep, which is where the body restores itself, regenerates for the next day, and keeps itself functioning smoothly (helpguide.org: How Much Sleep Do You Need?).

One of the most serious side effects of sleep apnea is an increased risk for heart complications. When you are not getting enough oxygen into your blood, your cardiovascular system is strained to keep fresh blood flowing through you. This increases your blood pressure and leaves you at risk to develop hypertension (continual high blood pressure). Untreated sleep apnea can lead to a detrimental and/or fatal heart incident (Mayo Clinic).

The lack of restorative sleep increases stress, which can put serious strain on the body. Continual stress will eventually affect every part of one's life, from health to relationships. On the outside you will start to notice muscle cramps, tension, or other pain; fatigue and lack of focus; chest pain; and declining sex drive. You are at risk of becoming anxious, restless, angry, irritable, and depressed. You may lack motivation to get through the day, complete tasks, or engage with others. Stress can lead to overeating, which can lead to weight gain and the negative health effects associated with it. It can also lead to undereating, substance abuse, defensive or angry behavior, and social withdrawal (Mayo Clinic).

Another issue is that a lack of sleep at night can increase the chances of you falling asleep during the day. This would be very dangerous while you were driving or operating machinery. It also would hinder your ability to effectively work and engage with others.

Sleep apnea can cause complications with surgery because you are less able to breath when lying on your back or under sedation. Before any medical procedure, make sure that you talk to your doctor about all of the possible complications, including your sleep apnea, so that they can find a solution best fit to your needs.

Diagnosing and Treating Sleep Apnea

Deciding whether or not to have yourself tested for sleep apnea can be difficult. You face the decision of having to take time off of work, potentially expensive medical bills, and the inconvenience of disrupting your daily schedule. None of those things are to be taken lightly—they are probably each very important to you. But leaving a serious condition undiagnosed and untreated can be very dangerous. Your sleep apnea can turn into something worse, like a heart condition from the added stress; or it can worsen an already existing condition. It is safest to consult a doctor about any problems you or a partner might notice.

Now, where is the line between normal sleeping with a few disruptions, and sleep apnea? Who has not snored, woken up during the night, or been tired in the morning? Sometimes normal things can explain away symptoms that might look like sleep apnea. For example, mild snoring can be caused by allergies, a weird sleep position, etc. We can be restless at night because we are stressed. We can have a hard time waking up or staying awake because we have had a long week at work or with the kids.

As defined by Doug Linder of New Technology Publishing, apnea can be described as any disturbance in the sleep. Sleep apnea as we are describing it is a chronic condition in which the sleep is repeatedly disturbed throughout the night. It should be treated if the pause in breathing is longer than 10 seconds at a time and/or you have more than 5 pauses per hour overnight. Less than 10 seconds at a time or less than 5 episodes in an hour is considered normal.

If you are not experiencing apnea with that much frequency, but you still feel like you are constantly exhausted and not getting healthy sleep, you can always talk to a doctor to see if perhaps you have another issue. It never hurts to check.

Here are some questions that you or a sleeping partner can answer to assess whether you should consider professional diagnosis:

- Do you snore loudly and frequently?
- Do you have pauses in breathing longer than 10 seconds while you sleep?
- Do you have heartburn at least twice a week?
- Do you suffer from insomnia (do you get up often without knowing why)?
- Are you restless while you sleep? Do you toss and turn all night?

- Do you assume a strange sleeping position? Do you need to be propped up every night to sleep properly?
- During the night, do you wake up gasping for breath, or with the feeling that you were just choking?
- Do you repeatedly jerk around in your sleep?
- Do you always wake up unalert and exhausted?
- Do you fall asleep during the day while doing something?
- Do you complete tasks in a daze, as if you cannot focus on them?
- Are you depressed, angry, irritable, or stressed for an unknown reason?

All of these can be symptoms of sleep apnea (New Technology Publishing). Sleep apnea can spread to other areas of your life, like causing you to be irritable or stressed, because of the way it interrupts your sleep. Since sleep is so vital to maintaining physical and mental health, your sleep apnea is a concern and should be treated accordingly.

<u>Breathing Devices for Sleep Apnea</u>

There are several options when it comes to treating sleep apnea. Surgery is not always necessary, or the most cost-effective means of treatment. One way to prevent sleep apnea is to use an oral device that is designed for those with obstructive sleep apnea, also called a mandibular repositioning device. This device is fitted like a retainer and it pushes the tongue and jaw forward.

The two main types of oral devices fall into either the tongue retaining appliances or the mandibular repositioning appliances categories. Tongue retaining appliances hold the tongue in place so that the base cannot sink down over the opening to the throat. Mandibular repositioning devices jut the lower jaw forward, keeping the muscles of the tongue tightened and preventing it from sinking back over the airway. Both of these help to increase air flow by keeping the airway open. There is less of a risk of the airway closing on itself while you are asleep. Oral devices are ideal for those who:

- Maintain a healthy weight
- Have mild to moderate sleep apnea
- Do not or cannot use a Continually Positive Airway Pressure (CPAP) treatment, although an oral device is usually not as effective as a CPAP treatment
- Tried other methods that failed, including behavior modification, other devices, or surgery

These devices have about a 50% success rate and are fitted and adjusted by a dentist or orthodontist. It is important to have them properly sized and to replace them should they become damaged in any way. They do have some drawbacks, though, that include:

- The device can cause an uncomfortable buildup of saliva.
- The device itself can become uncomfortable with the way that it positions your jaw or tongue, causing some people to ditch it in favor of a different solution.
- Misfitted devices can cause damage to your teeth, your gums, soft tissues in your mouth, or your jaw joints.
- These devices are not effective with central sleep apnea.

For consistent results, make sure that you wear your device every night. These devices can be preferred because they are light, discreet, and easy to travel with. They do not include any kind of surgery, so they can easily be removed during the day and are in no way an irreversible measure. Patients typically become used to the way they feel after a few weeks, lessening any discomfort (American Academy of Dental Sleep Medicine).

Oral Appliances for Sleep Apnea

Another method of treating sleep apnea without resorting to surgery is to use a Continuous Positive Airway Pressure system (called a CPAP). There are many different brands and models of CPAPs, but in general they provide a steady stream of air that keeps the airway open while one sleeps. This prevents the parts of the mouth from closing over the opening to the throat.

Treatment is administered by a CPAP machine that is comprised of a small device that blows air into a tube that connects to a mask secured to your head with an adjustable strap. The machine assists you in breathing all night and can be taken off in the morning. Some CPAP machines are more embellished and come with more features, like humidifiers. Manufacturers are moving toward a lightweight trend, and CPAPs can be found as small as 4x6.5 inches, weighing about 2 pounds. That's small enough to fit into the palm of your hand. Consequently, these are easy to transport and less bulky and conspicuous than before (cpap.com).

CPAPs apply a mild jet of air and are usually more effective than tongue retaining or mandibular repositioning devices. The machine itself is very quiet and usually emits nothing more than a rhythmic hum.

CPAPs are ideal for those who:

- Have moderate to severe sleep apnea
- Have not had success with other breathing devices
- Have mild to moderate sleep apnea
- Have central sleep apnea (as tongue retaining and mandibular repositioning devices are not effective in that case)
- Do not need or do not want to try surgery (National Heart, Lung, and Blood Institute)

There are some drawbacks to CPAPs, though:

- They can cause skin irritation or inflame through allergens. You can switch to a mask made of a different material, ask for a mask that has less skin contact, or even switch to a kind of CPAP that uses "nostril pillows," which are little inserts that you put into your nose.

- Using a CPAP can give you dry mouth. This could be because air is leaking from the mask, or you sleep with your mouth open to compensate for the sensation of the CPAP. In either case, you can consider getting a CPAP with a humidifier or a chin strap to keep your mouth closed.
- A leaking mask can also cause eye or skin irritation, or it can make an obnoxious sound as air is escaping.
- The constant air flow can cause problems with your sinuses, congestion, sneezing, or give you nosebleeds. Some people use nasal sprays to combat these effects. Also, always make sure that the mask is secure and not leaking.
- The air flow can cause stomach bloating or discomfort. It can also make one feel as if they cannot exhale, or cause them to feel like they are choking. Some CPAPs come with a "ramping" feature that allows the pressure to slowly increase to the needed levels, so the pressure is not all at once. Make sure to talk to a doctor and find a comfortable solution (National Heart, Lung, and Blood Institute).

Some general instructions that come with using a CPAP include:

1. Wash the mask and your face daily to prevent breakouts.
2. Use moisturizer to keep the mask from irritating your skin.
3. Get the right size mask and make sure that you secure it appropriately (not too tight, not too loose, as both can cause leaks).
4. Wear your sleep mask every night.

Your doctor will work with you to find the right settings that are just enough to meet your needs. Just as with brands and models, there are different styles of straps and mask materials that may be better suited for you. Be sure to keep communicating with your doctor about your needs and preferences so that you are getting the best product you can.

<u>Surgeries for Sleep Apnea</u>

Sometimes, people need to take more invasive measures to cure their sleep apnea. Always stay in close communication with a doctor about your need for a treatment, especially when it comes to surgery. Learn and consider each of the pros and cons before deciding to proceed with anything life-changing.

CPAP systems are often the first attempt at combating sleep apnea. But up to 50% of the time, patients have a hard time adjusting to them. They find the air pressure to be disconcerting or the masks uncomfortable. No system is going to be effective if the patient does not want to use it, so corrective surgeries may be the best option. The surgery selected should be tailored to the patient's specific needs, and can be performed on any part of the upper respiratory system (American Sleep Apnea Association).

The most common surgery of the last 25 years is called UPPP, or uvulopalatopharyngoplasty. In this procedure, a surgeon removes the tonsils (if present) and excess tissue around the pharynx and the soft palate. Sutures are inserted in the airway to keep it propped open. This procedure can cause pain for up to a week and requires an overnight hospital stay.

A less invasive procedure is a surgery that stiffens the soft palate. The soft palate implant, also known as the Pillar Procedure, is done by inserting three polyester rods into the soft palate. The rods cause a mild inflammatory reaction that stiffens the soft palate, making it more rigid. Since the palate is more rigid, it is less likely to fall down over the opening to the throat. Snoring is greatly reduced. This procedure can be done under local anesthesia while the patient is still alert (American Sleep Apnea Association).

Nasal surgery can cure problems in the nose that are related to sleep apnea. It consists of a septoplasty (surgery to repair a deviated septum, which is a displacement of the bone and cartilage in your nose that divides your two nostrils) and a turbinate reduction (Mayo Clinic). This surgery should straighten out the nasal cavity and reduce the size of turbinates (small sections inside the nostril) so that airflow is less constricted. Cartilage from the deviated septum can be removed and reinserted into the airway valve to prevent it from collapsing (American Rhinologic Society).

Hyoid advancement is a minimally invasive surgery that is gaining popularity among patients and surgeons. The hyoid is the bone that connects the tongue's muscles to the throat. Sometimes, people with sleep apnea have an enlarged tongue, or their tongue relaxes during sleep and obstructs their airway. The hyoid bone can be repositioned by butting a suture around it that pulls it forward toward the jaw. This procedure expands the airways and provides unobstructed air flow. The surgery can be completed in an hour, patients are free to leave afterward, and the pain is very minimal (American Sleep Apnea Association).

Genioglossus advancement is a similar surgery, in that it displaces the tongue to create better air flow. The genioglossus is the largest muscle in the tongue. A square section of the jaw is taken out, with the muscle attached, and moved forward in the mouth. The section is then reattached using a titanium plate. The plate has to be sturdy so that the muscle will not fall back into the base of the mouth. This procedure is effective, but it is much more invasive than the similar hyoid advancement, and it requires at least an overnight stay at the hospital.

Another method that alters the tongue is tongue base reduction surgery. It can be performed in two ways. The patient can undergo a series of radiofrequency treatments that are applied directly to the base of the tongue. They are designed to shrink the tongue tissue without causing damage to surrounding areas. Several treatments have to be performed before the method is effective. Another way to reduce the base of the tongue is to remove tissue using electrocautery or coblation (arthrocare.com). Both include using heat waves to reduce the tissue at the tongue's base (Medoscope). All of these methods are minimally invasive and can be done while the patient is awake, but doctors require patients to stay overnight to make sure that there are no adverse side effects (American Sleep Apnea Association).

An incredibly invasive but also incredibly effective procedure with a success rate of about 90% is lower jaw advancement. Sometimes the cause of sleep apnea is that someone is born with a naturally small jaw, which means they have a naturally restricted airway. Maxillomandibular advancement is a procedure in which the upper and lower jaws are expanded between 10 to 12 millimeters. The jaw is held in place with titanium plates. The jaw has to be held shut for several weeks so that it heals in the correct position. This is a precise and difficult procedure that several doctors and hospitals avoid doing because of the possibilities of complications. Bone cuts and teeth placement have to be precise so that the surgery is productive.

A tracheostomy is a procedure that is reserved for the morbidly obese. It is a permanent incision in the throat that provides direct access for air to enter the lungs. A structure that keeps the throat open and continually allows air flow is inserted, called a tracheostomy tube. Tracheostomies have their own complications, including accidental removal of the tube, infections in the trachea and around the tube, and damage to the throat that can arise from bacteria buildup, scar tissue from the surgery, or irritation or friction caused by the tube moving against the throat. This is an invasive surgery that is used as a last measure for when other methods have been tried and have failed (John Hopkins Medicine).

With sleep apnea in children, surgery to remove their tonsils or adenoids is often recommended. Some 75% of the time, this is an effective measure. Children may also be encouraged to lose weight, but they are much less likely to be encouraged to undergo surgery, especially anything severe because they are still developing. It is recommended that a speech-language pathologist referral be made for children prior to receiving surgery for adenoid removal for sleep apnea, as resonance in speech may be impacted by surgery.

Sometimes, surgeries to treat obesity are recommended to fix the underlying cause of the sleep apnea. There are a vast number of surgeries, therapies, and lifestyle changes available to lose weight, but one should talk to their doctor before making any major diet or lifestyle changes.

<u>Alternative Treatments and Home Remedies</u>

Sometimes, patients do not want to or cannot undergo any of the above treatments. Sleep apnea sufferers should always consult their doctors and make their needs and preferences very clear. Be sure to understand the outcome of each available course of action.

If you want to try something other than devices and surgery, you can undergo oxygen therapy. Doctors have mixed reviews on whether oxygen therapy should be used, so be sure to see what stance your doctor takes and do some research for yourself. In an article written by Brandon Peters, M.D., in February of 2014, he explains that, in some patients, oxygen therapy bettered their sleep apnea. The driving theory behind oxygen therapy is that increasing oxygen levels will solve the problem where patients cannot draw enough breath to oxygenate their blood. In theory, that makes sense. But in application, the results are all over the board. Pauses in breathing and daytime sleepiness are not affected, which are the main complaints of sleep apnea.

If the airway is not free of obstruction (as it often is not in obstructive sleep apnea), the oxygen has nowhere to go and your breathing can get worse. This leads to all sorts of things like dry mouth, headaches and disorientation. Oxygen may be an effective supplement to another treatment, but it probably will not bring you the desired relief by itself (Brandon Peters: Oxygen Therapy in Sleep Apnea).

In mild cases of sleep apnea, a patient may only need to undergo a few lifestyle changes to improve their symptoms. John Hopkins medicine recommends that you avoid alcohol, tobacco, and sleeping pills. Sleep on your side instead of on your back. If the head is tilted to the side or slightly downward, the walls and tongue are much less likely to close over the airway opening. Try to lose weight, even if it is only by 10% of your current weight. That amount of weight loss can have a great impact on clearing up your sleep apnea (John Hopkins Medicine).

Sometimes, self-treating sleep apnea may be the most effective method. Remember, though, that if you continually have problems with sleep apnea, it can lead to greater health problems. If you are not achieving desired results, it may be time to at least consult a physician to know where you stand. Here are a few ways that you can combat sleep apnea yourself:

-Lose your excess weight. As mentioned above, even a 10% decrease in body weight can mean a great improvement in your sleep apnea. This will reduce the pressure put on your neck, along with providing a vast array of other health benefits, and cessation of circumstances that could be putting unnecessary stress on your lungs and heart.

-Make sleep and exercise a priority. Both of these can combat the symptoms of sleep apnea. If you already are not getting the recommended amount of sleep, your sleep apnea will be worse. Exercise can also combat the negative effects of sleep apnea, like weight gain, stress, and moodiness.
-Limit your use of alcohol, and any drugs that are considered "downers" or tranquilizers. These relax your muscles, making it even easier for the muscles in your throat to collapse in on themselves, or fall back and block your airway.

-Do not sleep on your back. In that position it is easiest for your throat to be obstructed. Instead, sleep on your stomach or side. This will provide you with the best possible airflow.

-Quit smoking, as it is a cause of sleep apnea. Fluid from smoking builds around the lungs and puts pressure on your breathing.

Remember to always hold yourself to realistic expectations. If you are doing your best, but your sleep apnea persists, consider getting a professional evaluation. It could be that you have an uncontrollable disposition towards sleep apnea (such as your throat is naturally smaller than average) or that you have a sleep apnea that is not easily cured (possibly central sleep apnea).

In a study performed by Dr. Christopher P. Ward and six of his colleagues in 2009, they found that double reed musical instrument players are at less risk of developing obstructive sleep apnea. This is thought to occur because playing that type of instrument requires certain muscle movements that other wind instruments do not.

Another study done earlier had asserted that playing an instrument had no effect on whether a person developed obstructive sleep apnea. In 2008, Devin L. Brown of the University of Michigan published a study of 1,111 musicians who played a wide variety of instruments, from single reed, to double reed, to non-wind instruments. Brown asserted that musicians of any one instrument were no more likely to develop sleep apnea than any other instrument.

Ward's team's findings were different because they focused solely on the different types of wind instruments. In fact, they found that players of high pressure brass instruments like the trumpet and French horn are twice as likely to develop sleep apnea than double reed musicians. This group actually had the highest disposition towards obstructive sleep apnea in the entire survey. Single reed woodwind musicians (those who play flutes, clarinets, and saxophones), low-pressure brass musicians (those who play trombones and tubas) and non-wind instruments were strung somewhere in between the two extremes (American Sleep Apnea Association).

Sleep Apnea Wrap-up

Hopefully this book shed new light on the causes, symptoms, dispositions toward, and treatments of sleep apnea. Sleep apnea is a serious condition that is sometimes difficult to diagnose, but relatively easy to treat. There is no reason that you or a loved one should suffer through this disorder any longer. Consider the short- and long-term health risks associated with untreated sleep apnea, and consider what the best option is for you. Treatment does not always mean expensive surgeries or doctor appointments. It can start with simple at-home measures.

Consider these simple tips:

1. Keep a sleep diary for at least a week. Write down every time that you wake up. Ask your sleeping partner or housemates when they noticed you snoring, jolting awake, or choking. Be vigilant in recording how you feel during the day, any times that you unexpectedly fall asleep or nap, and what your stress level is.
2. For a variety of healthy reasons, make sleep a priority. Go to sleep at the same time and sleep for the recommended amount of time each night. Getting less than seven and a half to nine hours of sleep per night hinders your physical restoration and your mental development. It can leave you exhausted, unfocused, and lethargic. If you are getting the recommended amount of sleep but still having sleep apnea symptoms, consider different methods.
3. Maintain a healthy weight. In adults, obesity is the leading cause of obstructive sleep apnea—by far. Losing just a little weight can really clear up your symptoms. Try a combination of dieting and weight loss to get the desired effect. Hopefully, as you lose weight, your sleep apnea symptoms will lessen, and you will have more energy to be more physically active.
4. And, as always, do not be afraid to consult your doctor. Doctors are here to help you in the way that is best for you! You can work with them to find a realistic, affordable, desired solution to your sleep apnea.

You can be well on your way towards a life free of sleep apnea today. Consider your various options and settle on the one that combines the right health benefits and realistic expectations for you.

An Introduction to Diabetes

Diabetes is a complex illness that affects nearly 10% of all Americans. What is it? How does it affect the body? And, what can I do to prevent myself from getting diabetes or treat the diabetes that I already have? This book will answer each question in turn and give you a rich insight into this disease.

<u>What Is Diabetes?</u>

The simple definition of diabetes is "a metabolic disease in which the body's inability to produce any or enough insulin causes elevated levels of glucose in the blood" (Google define). Diabetes (or diabetes mellitus) is a group of conditions in which the patient has high blood sugar (a high concentration of glucose in the blood) because they do not produce enough insulin or their body does not respond properly to insulin. There could also be a combination of these two symptoms.

So, what is insulin? The standard definition is as such: "A hormone produced in the pancreas by the islets of Langerhans that regulates the amount of glucose in the blood. The lack of insulin causes a form of diabetes" (Google definition). In general, the hormone insulin is secreted from the pancreas when the body detects that there is sugar in the blood. There is sugar in your blood after you eat. Insulin is essential to balancing the amount of sugar (glucose) that you keep in your blood. When insulin is absent, you keep much more sugar in your blood than you are supposed to.

Diabetes can manifest itself in different ways, and it is a fast-spreading disease in the United States. There are three distinct types: type I diabetes, type II diabetes, and gestational diabetes. Type II diabetes is by far the most common, and gestational diabetes only occurs in pregnant women.

In 2012, 9.3% of Americans (nearly 10% of the population!), or 29.1 million people, had suffered from diabetes. The American Diabetes Association estimates that of that 29.1 million, 8.1 million were cases of people who had undiagnosed diabetes. Reported cases of diabetes were recorded by self-report means, while unreported cases of diabetes were found by testing for fasting glucose and hemoglobin A1C in subjects' blood samples (American Diabetes Association).

Since diabetes is such a dangerous diseases that can lead to other health issues, it is very important that it be diagnosed and treated as soon as possible. Diabetes is the seventh leading cause of death in the United States, as either the primary cause of death, the underlying cause of death, or the contributing cause of death.

In the next section there is a breakdown of each type of diabetes, who they affect, and how they specifically affect the body.

Diabetes Explained (I, II, and Gestational)

What is type I diabetes? In this type of diabetes, the body does not produce insulin. It can also be called "insulin-dependent diabetes," "early-onset diabetes," or "juvenile diabetes." This is because the subject is either born without the ability to produce insulin or loses the ability to produce insulin at a young age, usually during their teens or early adulthood. It is often not developed after someone's fortieth birthday, and only accounts for approximately 10% of all diabetic cases in the world (*Medical News Today*: What Is Diabetes? What Causes Diabetes?).

Those with type I diabetes will have to have insulin injections and eat a modified diet to balance their sugar intake for the rest of their lives. They will also have regular blood tests taken so that they can be sure that their bodies are maintaining proper glucose levels.

What is type II diabetes? This is a form of diabetes in which your body does not make enough insulin to manage your blood-glucose levels, or your cells do not react as they should to the insulin that is produced. This is also called "insulin resistance." This form of diabetes makes up the other 90% of cases worldwide.

Type II diabetes is developed later in life, for a variety of reasons. First, those who are overweight or obese are more at risk for developing type II diabetes. Those with an extreme amount of belly fat (also called visceral fat) or those labeled with central obesity are at even higher risk. Obesity can cause a person's body to release certain chemicals that work to throw the cardiovascular and metabolic systems out of rhythm.

Second, it is more prevalent in the elderly, for reasons that doctors and scientists do not quite understand. Their best conclusions determine that since we put on weight and become less active later in life, we are more at risk for contracting a disease that can be caused by these factors (*Medical News Today*: What Is diabetes? What Causes Diabetes?).

There are other leading causes—such as ethnicity and low testosterone levels in males—that directly contribute to type II diabetes. In general, it is believed to be a condition that is caused by putting on excess weight and not living an active lifestyle.

In 2012, the University of Edinburgh, United Kingdom, produced a study on mice that showed that low testosterone levels leave a subject at greater risk of developing type II diabetes. When the mice in the study did not have androgen receptors in their fat tissue (the receptors are what testosterone would attach itself to) they had greater insulin resistance than the mice who did have androgen receptors. The inability for testosterone to work effectively in the body, or when testosterone is not produced in adequate quantities, leaves a man at greater risk of resisting insulin and developing diabetes (*Medical News Today*: Men with Low Testosterone Levels May Be at Increased Risk for Diabetes).

In 2013, researchers at the Imperial College London, United Kingdom, conducted a study to determine if there was a link between sugary soft drink consumption and diabetes in Europe. In their study, researchers worked with approximately 350,000 volunteers from 8 countries: the United Kingdom, Italy, Spain, Germany, Denmark, France, Sweden, and the Netherlands. The study took into account all types of artificially sweetened drinks, including soft drinks, juices, and nectars. Findings showed that consuming only 12 ounces of a sugar drink each day increased the possibility of developing type II diabetes by 22% (*Medical News Today*: One Soda a Day Can Increase Diabetes Risk by 22%).

Similar studies have been done in the United States. Several studies were conglomerated together and a synopsis of their findings was published in a 2007 issue of the *American Journal of Public Health.* The project was supported by the Rudd Foundation, which is a private philanthropic organization that focuses on raising education about obesity. In one specific study, 91,249 women participated in a study that followed their eating habits for 8 years. The set of participants that consumed at least one soft drink per day were two times as likely to develop type II diabetes than those who only drank one soft drink per month or less (*Medical News Today*: Strong Evidence Links Soft Drink Consumption to Obesity, Diabetes).

Type II diabetes is often caused by obesity and sedentary lifestyles. Thus, it can be positively influenced by someone improving their diet and exercising.

What is gestational diabetes? This exclusively affects females during pregnancy, and usually goes away after childbirth—although it can leave women at greater risk for developing type II diabetes, and can leave the child at greater risk of being obese and developing type II diabetes.

Gestational diabetes is caused when a woman produces too much glucose during pregnancy and the body cannot handle it all. Normally, the body would take the blood glucose (sugar) and turn it into energy for the mother and unborn child to use. If too much is produced, though, the body cannot make enough insulin to take care of all that blood sugar, so the sugar stays in the blood.

Having this type of diabetes means that the pregnant woman is at greater risk of developing high blood pressure during pregnancy, and it could increase the chances of her needing to undergo a cesarean section versus a natural birth. A child born to a mother with gestational diabetes is at risk for being born large, with extra fat—which complicates the baby's delivery and postpartum health (National Healthy Mothers, Healthy Babies Coalition: Prenatal Monitoring and Care; The Lasting Impact of Gestational Diabetes on Mothers & Children).

Women who had a diet high in animal fat and cholesterol before becoming pregnant are at greater risk of developing gestational diabetes. Blood sugar levels usually return to normal for the mother after birthing her child, but she has a 35 to 60% greater chance of developing type II diabetes later in life. As with type II diabetes, gestational diabetes can be combated by eating a healthy diet and exercising regularly (*Medical News Today*: What Is Diabetes? What Causes Diabetes?).

How Diabetes Affects Your Body and Health, Directly and Indirectly

Your cells need two things to function: oxygen and sugar. Oxygen and sugar travel through your bloodstream to each cell. Once at the cells, oxygen is absorbed immediately. Sugar, however, needs insulin to help it permeate the cell. When you eat, your body naturally detects how much insulin you are going to need to accommodate that meal, and that much is ten excreted from the pancreas. Diabetics' bodies cannot accurately detect how much insulin is needed. That is why they have to take injections of insulin to sustain their blood sugar levels. They must be careful, though, because not enough insulin will leave the blood sugar high, while too much will cause it to plummet unhealthily.

Diabetes affects different people in different ways. Its effects vary by the three different types. Prolonged diabetes can also lead to other serious health issues. Some of the effects include the following:

Hypoglycemia: Hypoglycemia is the condition that occurs when a person's blood sugar is too low. This is a condition that only diabetics can have, although some of the symptoms may be seen in non-diabetic patients. Some of the medications that diabetic patients use to treat their diabetes have the adverse effect of lowering blood sugar. Blood sugar can also drop during prolonged periods of fasting (when someone is not eating), such as when you first wake up.

People use sugar as an energy source. If someone has not eaten for a long time, the body will naturally conserve glucose in the liver as glycogen. Once the sugar is needed, the body goes through a process called gluco-neo-genesis ("make new sugar") that extracts the glycogen and turns it back into usable sugar. The brain is the organ that depends on sugar for almost all of its nutrients (it can use ketones as a source of energy, but prefers not to). It does not have the ability to make its own sugar, so it relies almost completely on the metabolic system for its energy (http://www.medicinenet.com/hypoglycemia/article.htm: Hypoglycemia).

Normal levels of sugar are in the 70–100 mg/dL range before breakfast. When the body senses that blood sugar is falling below these levels, it has measures to protect itself. It enacts a series of hormones (glucagon, epinephrine, and cortisol) that work to raise blood sugar. It stops creating insulin, which would normally lower blood sugar. The body will then send signals to the person that manifest themselves as symptoms of hypoglycemia.

When a person's blood sugar is in the mid- to high 70s mg/dL, the body starts to release its stores of glycogen and enacts the other hormones. Usually, people will not have any symptoms in this stage.

Patients start feeling the first set of symptoms when their blood sugar drops below 50 mg/dL. These are the nervous system's response to the drop in glucose, and they are called adrenergic or sympathetic. They include intense hunger, sweating, nervousness, trembling, weakness, palpitations, and trouble with speech.

These symptoms are the body's way of alerting itself to the need to eat, which will raise blood sugar. An episode can typically be overcome once the person eats. If a person does not or cannot eat, their condition progresses. They move from having nervous system symptoms to having neuro-glyco-penic symptoms, meaning that their blood sugar levels are affecting brain function. These symptoms include confusion, behavioral changes, drowsiness, coma, and/or seizure.

It is very important to treat hypoglycemia quickly, whenever it happens. This can be done by eating or drinking sugary foods or drinks. At first, a hypoglycemic episode should be treated with 15 grams of sugar. That is approximately four teaspoons of sugar, four lifesavers candies, one half of a can of soft drink, or one half of a can of fruit juice.

If the symptoms do not subside in the next 10 minutes, another 10–15 grams should be consumed. This cycle can be repeated three times. If there is no improvement after the third try, the patient is considered non-responsive and professional medical assistance should be acquired.

In 2011, approximately 282,000 cases of emergency room visits for adults 18 years old or older cited hypoglycemia as the leading cause of emergency, with diabetes as a secondary diagnosis.

Hyperglycemia: Hyperglycemia occurs when the body's blood sugar levels get too high (as opposed to hypoglycemia, when they are too low). It is most commonly caused by diabetes, although it can be caused by a few other illnesses, including pancreatitis, pancreatic cancer, Cushing's syndrome, and tumors that are excreting unusual hormones.

Normal levels of sugar are in the 70–10 mg/dL range before breakfast. They are higher after eating, but at regular intervals during the day they should be less than 125 mg/dL. When blood sugar levels are elevated much beyond that, the result can be a serious medical emergency. High blood sugar can lead to diabetic ketoacidosis (DKA) or hyperglycemic hyperosmolar nonketotic syndrome (HHNS) (http://www.medicinenet. com/hyperglycemia/article.htm: Hyperglycemia). Diabetic ketoacidosis affects people with type I diabetes, while hyperglycemic hyperosmolar nonketotic syndrome affects people with type II diabetes (http://www.medicinenet.com/ hyperglycemia/page3.htm).

Long-term untreated high blood sugar can lead to a host of other maladies, because of the damage that it does to blood vessels (http://www.medicinenet.com/diabetic_ ketoacidosis_symptoms/views.htm: Diabetic Ketoacidosis Symptoms). These complications include stroke, kidney failure, heart attack, amputations, and/or blindness.

From 2005–2008, in adult cases of patients who were 40 years old or older and who suffered from diabetes, 4.2 million of them had diabetic retinopathy (that is, 28.5%). Diabetic retinopathy is a condition in which the long-term effects of diabetes cause damage to the blood vessels, specifically those small vessels in the retina. This damage can impair and/or cause loss of vision (http://www.diabetes.org/diabetes-basics /statistics/).

In 2010, the rate of patients hospitalized for stroke was one and a half times higher for the diabetic community as it was for those who are not diagnosed with diabetes. Hospitalization rates for heart attacks in adult diabetics was 1.8 times higher than it was for those who were not diabetic.

Also in 2010, approximately 73,000 non-traumatic lower-limb amputations were undergone by adult patients who were diagnosed with diabetes. This means that approximately 60% of non-traumatic, lower-limb amputations performed on adults were in adults that were diagnosed with diabetes (http://www.diabetes.org/diabetes-basics/statistics/).

In 2011, 44% of all new cases of kidney failure listed diabetes as the primary cause. That year, almost 50,000 people (children and adults) began treatment for kidney failure due to diabetes. In 2011, a little less than 300,000 people (children and adults) with kidney failure resulting from diabetes participated in chronic dialysis or had a kidney transplant (http://www.diabetes.org/diabetes-basics/statistics/).

Diabetic ketoacidosis happens when your body's cells cannot absorb sugar from the blood because of a lack of insulin. Since your body cannot get nutrients from sugar (since the sugar you eat cannot be absorbed), it turns to fat as an alternative fuel source. Breaking down fat is not very healthy, though, because it releases toxic acids called ketones. These acids build up in the bloodstream. This is a fatal condition if left untreated, so be cautious when checking for symptoms (Mayo Clinic: Diabetic Ketoacidosis). They include frequently needing to urinate, being excessively thirsty, becoming nauseated and/or vomiting, pain in the abdomen, weakness, shortness of breath, fatigue, confusion, and/or "fruit-scented" breath.

You can check yourself at home by checking to see if your blood sugar is higher than your normal range, using an over-the-counter ketone testing kit. See a doctor if either of your tests is abnormally high (for ketone tests, that means if your ketone levels are moderate to high) or if you are vomiting and cannot keep down food or liquids (Mayo Clinic: Diabetic ketoacidosis, When to see a doctor).

In hyperglycemic cases, sugar can be detected in the blood. This does not normally happen because the body should absorb all the sugar that is ingested. Other symptoms of hyperglycemia include severe thirst, needing to urinate often, headaches, blurred vision, exhaustion, hunger, and/or difficulty concentrating or comprehending.

In 2011, approximately 175,000 visits to the emergency room by adults had hyperglycemic crisis as the first diagnosis.

<u>Diabetes Demographics</u>

Does diabetes affect different groups of the population differently? Who is most at risk, and which group—whether by race or age—has the greatest predisposition towards developing diabetes?

According to the National Diabetes Statistics Report 2014, American Indians/Alaskan natives are the group that has the highest rate of diabetes reports by population (American Diabetes Association: Statistics About Diabetes). Below is a chart depicting the percent of diabetic cases broken down by ethnicity.

American Indians/Alaskan natives: 15.9%
Non-Hispanic African Americans: 13.2%
Hispanics: 12.8%
Asian Americans: 9.0%
Non-Hispanic Caucasians: 7.6%

(Information taken from the National Diabetes Statistics Report, 2014)

While all humans have the same basic makeup, there are obviously disparities between races when it comes to how much of the population develops diabetes. Leroy M. Graham, Jr. MD contributes to an article published on WebMd that tries to explain some of these differences. Graham is a pediatric lung specialist and an associate clinical professor of pediatrics at Morehouse School of Medicine in Atlanta. He serves on the American Lung Association's board of directors, and as staff physician for Children's Healthcare of Atlanta.

Graham explains that, first, there could be genetic differences between races that predispose some to be more susceptible to diseases. This assertion is taken from several statistics: 60% more African Americans have diabetes than Caucasians. Fatal lung scarring is 16 times more likely to occur in African Americans than Caucasians. African American men are 50% more likely to get lung cancer than Caucasians, even though they report lower tobacco use than Caucasians. And, fatal strokes are four times more likely in African Americans than Caucasians in the 35- to 54-year-old category (WebMD: Health care disparities heighten disease differences between African-Americans and white Americans).

Clyde W. Yancy, MD is an associate dean of clinical affairs and the director for heart failure and transplants at the University of Texas Southwestern Medical Center. Doctor Yancy says that everyone has the same physical makeup   we are all vulnerable to the same diseases, and respond the same to medicines. While this is true on a fundamental level, there are certain other factors that put some people at greater health risks.

Those factors include education, location of where you live and work, and access to health care. Living in an area that is exposed to toxic waste dumping, factories that expel toxic waste, or places that violate federal standards for emissions and air pollution would put you at greater risk of developing lung cancer and all the associated health issues. Also, not being diagnosed and treated in the early stages of your disease can lead to greater complications and fatality rates. This factor would relate to any disease, from diabetes to heart failure. Education is the factor that ties the other two together. In families or communities that do not understand the importance of screenings and preventative treatment, people are more likely to be diagnosed later in the life of their diseases. That limits their treatment options and gives the disease time to spread to other areas of their body, allowing it to affect their health more (WebMD:Health care disparities heighten disease differences between African-Americans and white Americans).

Rates of Diabetes Are Also Broken Down by Age:

In adults 18 to 44 years old, there are 3,392,000 people who have diabetes. That is 15.8% of the United States' diabetic population and 3.1% of the United States' overall population. In adults 45 to 64 years old, there are 9,765,000 people who have diabetes. That is 45.5% of the United States' diabetic population and 12.3% of the United States' overall population. In adults 65 to 74 years old, there are 4,624,000 people who have diabetes. That is 21.5% of the United States' diabetic population and approximately 6% of the United States' overall population. In adults 75 years old and older, there are 3,684,000 people who have diabetes. That is 17.2% of the United States' diabetic population and approximately 4.5% of the United States' overall population.

(This data taken from the United States Census 2010 and the State Health Fact sheet that was published by The Henry J. Kaiser Family Foundation. This data was extrapolated from the United States Census 2010 and the State Health Facts published by The Henry J. Kaiser Family Foundation, using the following formula: In the 2010 Census, total United States population for the age group 65 years plus equaled 40,267,984. In the Kaiser Foundation publication, this group was broken into two subgroups: 65–74 years old and 75 plus years old. The number of total diabetics for the two groups were added together (8,308,000) and divided by the total population for the two groups (40,267,984), equaling 20.6% of the United

States population. This number (20.6%) was divided on a 60/40 basis, with the 65-to 74-year-old group maintaining 60% and the 75 plus group maintaining 40%.)

Another interesting statistic is the breakdown of what age someone is first diagnosed at. The Center for Disease Control and Prevention provides that breakdown here:

18–29 years old: 4.3%
30–34 years old: 4.5%
35–39 years old: 6.8%
40–44 years old: 8.9%
45–49 years old: 10.9%
50–54 years old: 14.2%
55–59 years old: 15.4%
60–64 years old: 13.8%
65–69 years old: 9.5%
70–74 years old: 7.1%
75–79 years old: 4.7%

(Information taken from the Center for Disease Control and Prevention: Distribution of Age at Diagnosis of Diabetes Among Adult Incident Cases Aged 18–79 Years, United States, 2011.)

While no one can change their predisposition towards diabetes, it can certainly be warded off by taking particular health measures. If you think you suffer from diabetes, or have any of the preceding symptoms, please see a physician as soon as possible. They can use blood tests to determine the health issues you may or may not have. Early detection and prevention are crucial to keeping diabetes in check. The longer you wait, the worse your condition will become.

<u>Maintaining a Healthy Weight: Fat, Protein, and Carbohydrates Explained</u>

All food is made up of calories. Calories are measures of energy, so when we eat we are consuming energy to get through our day. In recent years, scientists and nutritionists have learned that not all calories are "made equal." This means that 100 calories of sweets will not affect you the same way that 100 calories of eggs will. The makeup of calories is very important in understanding what is healthy and what is not.

There are two competing theories in the health world: Is it better to eat a diet low in fat or low in carbohydrates to lose weight? For a while, people intuitively assumed that it would be better to eat a diet lower in fat. Now, however, several studies have come out showing that eating a diet lower in carbohydrates will help you lose weight faster. Some of these include:

1. Samaha FF trial of a low-carb diet for severe obesity, published in the *New England Journal of Medicine* 2003

In this trial, 132 severely obese individual (average BMI of 43) were divided randomly into an LC and an LF group. The LF dieters were calorie restricted. Many of these participants suffered from obesity-related diseases such as metabolic syndrome and type II diabetes. The study ran for six months.

The LC group lost more weight. The LF group lost an average of 4.2 pounds, while the LC group lost 12.8 pounds—three times as much! Other factors also leaned in favor of the LC group. Triglycerides and fasting blood glucose went down by 38 mg and 26 mg respectively in the LC group, but only 7 mg and 5 mg in the LF group. Insulin levels went down by 27% in the LC group, but slightly increased in the LF group. Also, insulin sensitivity improved in the LC group, but slightly increased in the LF group.

2. Sondike SB trial of a low-carb diet for overweight adolescents, *The Journal of Pediatrics* 2003

This trial studied 30 overweight adolescents divided into an LC and an LF group for 12 weeks. Neither group had to restrict their calories. The study found that the LC group lost 21.8 pounds and the LF group lost 9 pounds—a significant difference. The LC group also had significant decreases in triglycerides and non-HDL cholesterol.

From these studies we can see that a diet low in carbs is better for losing weight. So, why are carbohydrates worse than fat? One reason is that different calories affect your metabolism and hormones in different ways.

When you consume carbohydrates, your body breaks them down into sugar. This raises your blood sugar levels, which tells the pancreas to secrete enough insulin to lower your blood sugar levels. In Type II diabetics, the body has consumed so many sugar-producing foods (sweets, carbs) that the insulin-producing cells have worn out and stopped working. The result? Blood sugar is constantly high (Harvard School of Public Health: Carbohydrates and Blood Sugar).

Protein, on the other hand, is a metabolic stimulant. Approximately 30% of the calories consumed from protein are burned just in the digestion process. Protein works to suppress your appetite and boost your metabolism, which in turn burns more calories. Protein also builds up muscles, which are metabolic tissues that burn calories by themselves (Authority Nutrition).

Diabetic patients are often told not to eat meats, because the fat can raise their cholesterol, and they are already prone to heart complications. Lean meats, however, are a great alternative. They provide the needed protein that works with the metabolism, but they do not have so much unhealthy fat in them.

Lifestyle Changes to Undo Diabetes

Type I diabetes is not a reversible condition. The best thing to do is control your blood sugar levels, as instructed by your doctor. Type II diabetes, however, can sometimes be "reversed" by correcting the conditions that first caused the diabetes. High blood sugar levels can be detected early, and you can undergo some lifestyle changes (mostly modifications to diet and activity levels) to naturally reverse your diabetes symptoms.

The important thing, when considering major lifestyle changes, is to consult with your physician. Make sure that the changes you want to make coincide with what is best for your health. Some changes a doctor may suggest to a diabetic patient are to eat a healthy diet and be more active.

A healthy diet is important in keeping your blood sugar levels down. Becoming more active is important when it comes to losing weight and relieving some of your diabetic symptoms. For your diet, it is important to eat foods that are low in sugar and "simple" carbohydrates. Simple carbohydrates are carbs that absorb easily into the blood, therefore raising blood sugar levels very quickly. "Complex" carbs (defined as more than three sugars linked together) take longer for the body to breakdown, therefore taking longer to raise blood sugar levels (Harvard Public Health).

This easy method of dividing carbs into two categories has been replaced with a more realistic system that ranks carb from 0–100. This system is called the glycemic index. A higher number on the index means that the carb is absorbed faster than a lower number carb is.

Here are four low carb or "complex carb" foods (glycemic index less than 55):

Unsweetened oatmeal, barley, or other whole grains. Whole grains are better for you than white flour, because they are supposed to be less refined. The less refined it is, the harder it is to digest and the longer it takes your blood sugar to go up.

Green and/or leafy vegetables, like broccoli, spinach, and green beans. These foods are high in fiber and low in carbs, so they take longer to digest.

Lean meats such as skinless chicken breast, salmon and other fish, and venison. These provide protein to boost the metabolism, but have much less fat than other meats.

Water. As always, water is essential to any diet. Replace sugary sodas and teas with glasses of water. It has a myriad of health benefits, including helping you feel fuller and eat less (Mayo Clinic: Create your healthy eating plan).

Eating a specific diet can become difficult and frustrating at times, especially if you feel like you are restricted to just a few options. We are going to provide you with a week's worth of meal ideas, to give you a starting point with your diet. Remember to talk to your doctor before making major diet and lifestyle changes to make sure that they will have the desired effect for you.

Everyone requires a certain amount of calories to get through their day, called a base metabolic rate. Weight loss should be done slowly, so as to not throw the metabolism off balance. There is no sense in eating vastly less than you need to, because that triggers the "survival" instinct your body has to store fat and sugar, causing you to gain weight and ruining your metabolism.

This is a meal plan based on someone who needs approximately 1,500 calories a day. You may need more calories than this, so work with your doctor on a suitable meal schedule that meets your calorie needs. This chart will give you some ideas of healthy food choices. You can also use any online calorie counter, such as the great one found at www.calorieking.com, to get a rough estimate of your base metabolic rate.

Monday

Breakfast will consist of 1 cup of water, ½ of a whole grain bagel spread with 1 teaspoon of fruit spread and 1 teaspoon of cream cheese, and 1 cup of milk.

Lunch will consist of 1 cup or more of water, 2 cups of mixed dark greens (kale, spinach, lettuce), cucumbers, tomatoes, onion to taste, ½ cup garbanzo beans, 1 ounce of shredded cheese, and 2 tablespoons of light dressing.

Dinner will consist of 1 cup or more of water. Grill or roast 1 skinless chicken breast until cooked through. Top with 2 tablespoons of barbecue sauce. For coleslaw, mix 1 cup of shredded red and green cabbage, carrots, and 1 tablespoon of coleslaw dressing (or 2 tablespoons of low fat dressing). Serve on 1 slice of whole grain wheat toast or 1 slice of garlic sourdough toast. Spread bread with 1 tablespoon olive oil and garlic. Top bread with coleslaw.

Drink at least 1 more cup of water before bed.

Tuesday

Breakfast will consist of 1 cup of water, 6 ounces of light yogurt, ¼ cup of granola cereal, 1 tablespoon of ground flaxseed, 1 tablespoon of chopped nuts, cinnamon for taste (cinnamon is thought to have an insulin-like effect that lowers blood sugar), and 1 cup of milk.

Lunch will consist of 1 cup or more of water. Combine 2 cups of mixed dark greens (spinach, kale, lettuce), 2 stalks of celery, and ¼ cup of sliced green or red grapes. Top combination with 2 ounces of cooked chicken breast. Drizzle with 2 tablespoons of light honey mustard dressing. Serve on 1 slice of whole grain wheat toast. Spread toast with 1 tablespoon of butter.

Dinner will consist of 1 cup or more of water, 3–4 slices of lean roast beef (or 3 ounces), 1 cup cooked brown rice with seasonings to taste, and 1 cup cooked spinach, seasoned with 1 teaspoon of olive oil and 1 teaspoon of balsamic vinegar.

Drink at least 1 more cup of water before bed.

Wednesday

Breakfast will consist of 1 cup of water, 6 ounces of light yogurt, 2 tablespoons of dried fruit, 2 tablespoons of ground flaxseed, 2 tablespoons of chopped nuts, and 1 cup of milk.

Lunch will consist of 1 cup or more of water. Bake 1 corn tortilla at 400 degrees F in oven until crispy, then remove and spread with ½ cup cooked pinto beans and 2 tablespoons of cheese. Bake for 5–10 more minutes, or until cheese is melted. Remove and top with ¼ cup salsa. Shred 1 cabbage and mix with 1 chopped tomato for salad. Top salad with 2 tablespoons of low fat dressing.

Dinner will consist of 1 cup or more of water, 1 cup cooked whole grain pasta tossed with 1 tablespoon of olive oil and garlic, and 3 ounces of lean meat cooked into meatballs (turkey, chicken or soy). Sprinkle with 1 teaspoon of grated Parmesan cheese. For salad, combine 1 cup of mixed greens (spinach, kale, or lettuce), 1 cup of cucumber slices, 10 halved cherry tomatoes, and ¼ cup of chopped red onions. Top salad with 2 tablespoons of low fat dressing

Drink at least 1 more cup of water before bed.

Thursday

Breakfast will consist of 1 cup of water and 1 egg cooked with canola, peanut, or olive oil. Combine ½ cup of spinach and ½ cup of mushrooms, onion, garlic, and other herbs to taste. Top omelet with 2 tablespoons of cheese. Serve with 1 slice of whole grain wheat toast spread sparingly with butter, and 1 cup milk.

Lunch will consist of 1 cup or more of water, 2 whole grain wheat bread slices, 3 slices (approx. 2 ounces) of roast beef, 1 or 2 leaves of lettuce (or proportional amounts of spinach or kale), and ½ of a tomato (sliced). Top with 1 teaspoon of mayo or mustard.

Dinner will consist of 1 cup or more of water. Combine ⅓ cup of cooked brown rice with 2 tablespoons of crumbled feta cheese, scoop combination onto 2 cups of mixed greens, top with 3 ounces (or 1 handful) of grilled or sautéed shrimp (cook in olive oil), and drizzle with 2 tablespoons of low fat dressing. Serve with 1 slice of whole grain wheat toast spread with 2 tablespoons of butter, margarine, or cottage cheese.

Drink at least 1 more cup of water before bed.

Friday

Breakfast will consist of 1 cup of water, 1 apple cut into slices mixed with ½ cup of light yogurt, and 1 cup of milk.

Lunch will consist of 1 cup or more of water, 2 leaves of lettuce laid side by side and topped with 1 slice of any flavor cheese, 2 slices of ham sandwich meat, and 2 slices of turkey breast sandwich meat. Place the meat on top of the lettuce and roll up in such a way that the lettuce holds the contents together.

Dinner will consist of 1 cup or more of water. Toss 1 skinless chicken breast with 1 tablespoon of low fat Italian dressing or olive oil. Coat chicken and dressing in 2 tablespoons of Italian seasoned bread crumbs. Spray lightly with canola oil. Cook on tinfoil or highly oiled cookie sheet in the oven at 350 degrees F for 30 minutes, or until cooked through and the crumbs are golden brown. Mix ½ cup of green beans, ¼ cup of garbanzo beans, and ¼ cup of red beans with 2 tablespoons of chopped onion and a handful of lettuce or other leafy greens. Drizzle salad with 2 tablespoons of low fat dressing or olive oil.

Drink at least 1 more cup of water before bed.

Saturday

Breakfast will consist of 1 cup of water. Scramble 1 egg in pan sprayed with canola, peanut, or olive oil. Combine ¼ cup of chopped tomato, onion, and chili salsa into omelet. Serve with toasted whole grain wheat English muffin spread with 2 tablespoons cottage cheese, and 1 cup of milk.

Lunch will consist of 1 cup or more of water. Toss 1 ½ cups of broccoli heads lightly in olive oil with garlic, salt and pepper. Bake broccoli at 400 degrees F for 20–25 minutes, until edges are dark. Spread 1 skinless chicken breast with desired spices and olive oil. Bake chicken at 350 degrees F for 15–25 minutes, until cooked all the way through.

Dinner will consist of 1 cup or more of water. Coat 2 fish fillets with garlic, salt, pepper, and other seasonings to taste. Cook on stove in pan on medium to medium-high heat until the fish is thoroughly cooked through. Serve with 1 cup cooked whole grain brown rice.

Drink at least 1 more cup of water before bed.

Sunday

Breakfast will consist of 1 cup of water, ½ whole grain wheat bagel spread with 1 tablespoon cream cheese, and 1 cup of milk.

Lunch will consist of 1 cup or more of water and 2 halves of a whole grain English muffin. Top each half with 1 tablespoon of pesto basil sauce, 1 slice of tomato, and 1 slice of cheese. Bake in oven until cheese is melted.

Dinner will consist of 1 cup or more of water. Foil-bake 3 ounces of halibut (or other fish) with 1 cup of chopped green peppers and onions. Season with less than 1 teaspoon of olive oil and other seasonings to taste. Roast ½ cup of red potato chunks in 1 tablespoon of olive oil and season with herbs and spices to taste.

Drink at least 1 more cup of water before bed.

Snack options throughout the week are as follows:

1 orange and 1 small handful of almonds

1 banana

1 cup of fresh strawberries and 1 handful of unsalted nuts

1 cup of melon (watermelon, honeydew, cantaloupe) with 6 ounces of yogurt

1 kiwi and 1 small handful of almonds

1 medium apple with 2 tablespoons peanut butter

Celery stalks (as many as desired) with 2 tablespoons of peanut butter

5 dried apricot halves and 7 walnut halves

2 graham crackers spread with 1 tablespoon of all natural peanut butter

3 cups of lightly buttered popcorn and 16 ounces of light-sugar lemonade

¼ cup of cashews, almonds, or walnuts

4 vanilla wafers and 1 cup of milk

6 ounces of yogurt with ¾ cup of blueberries, blackberries, raspberries, or strawberries

½ cup of light ice cream

(Some meal ideas taken from Prevention.com: Outsmart Diabetes 5-Week Meal Plan.)

In addition to following a healthy diet, exercise and physical activity is important to work towards your progress. Talk to a doctor about what is right for you. It may be as simple as taking a brisk walk every day to get your heart up. For this, you can use a walking tracker like the FitBit Pedometer to track how far you have walked. The FitBit can come in different styles that you can either wear around your wrist or drop into your pocket. On top of counting your steps, it will also track how far you've walked and how many calories you've burned. At night it can track your sleeping habits and act as an alarm clock.

How to Stay Motivated and Track Your Progress

An important key to staying motivated and making progress towards your goals is to be realistic in your expectations and leave room for error. Do not be so stringent with your diet that you do not leave room for healthy snacks or slip-ups, because slip-ups are going to happen. It will be much more detrimental to you reaching your goal if you beat yourself up over every mistake. Instead, understand that every step made in the right direction is progress. Life changes do not occur overnight, so be patient and carefully track your progress. Tracking your progress is one of the best ways to see how far you've come, especially when you first start a new diet (because physical evidence is not always very clear).

To stay motivated, we suggest that you do two other things. The first is to find a friend or mentor that you can confide your goals in. Make sure that you are very clear with them about where you stand right now and where you want to be in a specified amount of time. This can be someone you live with who is going to modify their diet with you; a friend or coworker who is going to start exercising with you; or really anyone else that you trust. Regularly update this person on your progress. They will be invaluable in encouraging you when things are going well and picking you up should you stray from your goals.

The second thing is to keep a strict food journal. This is very important because we can sometimes overlook what we are eating. Writing everything down keeps us accountable to ourselves. Check out www.fitday.com for an easy-to-use online food journal. Or simply get a notebook and record the times you eat and what you eat to get a better grasp on your nutritional habits. This will give you a great idea of your patterns and where you can make adjustments and improvements.

In your journal, you can go as far as explaining how you feel each day, your current weight, and the breakdown of the foods by calories, carbs, etc. Over time, you can look for trends in the correlation between food and energy level or mood, and you will know exactly how many calories you consumed and what their makeup was.

Using a tool like the FitBit is a great way to see how much exercise you are getting. You can include this information in your food journal, along with all the things you ate that day and how you felt.

Medications

People with type I diabetes are going to have to take insulin. People with type II diabetes may be able to control their blood sugar through lifestyle changes. If not, they may also need insulin injections (if their bodies cannot make their own insulin). Figuring out the best type of insulin will involve a conversation with your doctor about what fits your needs. Basically, you can chose from fast-acting insulin, short-acting insulin, intermediate-acting insulin, long-acting insulin, and pre-mixed insulin.

How will your doctor determine what is best for you to use? That answer depends on many variables, including your age, your goals, how you respond to insulin (how long it takes your body to absorb the insulin), lifestyle choices (such as the types of food you eat, your alcohol consumption, and your activity level), your tolerance for insulin injections, and/or how often you are going to check your blood sugar levels.

Below are different insulin medications broken down by type. Discuss these options with a doctor to figure out which would suit you best.

Fast-acting:
Humalog or lispro, starts working in 15–30 minutes, lasts 3–5 hours
Novolog or aspart, starts working in 20 minutes, last up to 5 hours
Apidra or glulisine, starts working in 30 minutes, lasts up to 2.5 hours

Short-acting:
Regular ® humulin or novolin, starts working in less than an hour, last up to 8 hours
Velosulin, starts working in less than an hour, last up to 3 hours

Intermediate-acting:
NPH(N), starts working in less than 2 hours, last up to 24 hours

Long-acting:
Lantus, starts working between 1–1 ½ hours, last up to 24 hours
Levemir, starts working in 1–2 hours, last up to 24 hours

Pre-mixed (contains proportions of intermediate- and short-acting insulin):
Humulin 70/30, starts working in 30 minutes, last between 14–24 hours

Novolin 70/30, starts working in 30 minutes, last up to 24 hours
Novolog 70/30, starts working in 20 minutes, last up to 24 hours
Humulin 50/50, starts working in 30 minutes, last between 18–24 hours
Humalog mix 75/25, starts working in 15 minutes, last between 16–20
hours

(Information taken from http://www.webmd.com/diabetes/guide/diabetes-types-insulin.)

Diabetes Wrap-up

Diabetes can be a manageable condition. It is very helpful if symptoms are detected early, so that medication and lifestyle changes can have the greatest effect. Below are a few tips that summarize the suggestions given thus far:

Talk to your doctor! Work with them to decide what medication you need and what changes you need to make. They can tell you if a goal is too far-fetched for your current situation, which is always better to learn at the outset (instead of getting frustrated with what seems like slow progress).

Set realistic goals for exercise and dieting. Nothing is more frustrating than continually missing goals, so don't set yourself up for failure.

Find an "accountability partner." This can be anyone that you trust to tell about your condition and track your progress with you. They should be very helpful in encouraging your efforts and keeping you on track.

Keep a lifestyle journal. Be vigilant in recording everything you eat, every day. Having it all laid out on paper makes your progress very clear.

Part Four – Heart Disease

An Introduction to Heart Disease

Heart disease is a serious condition that should be diagnosed and treated by a licensed professional as soon as possible. Initial symptoms can lead to elevated risk the longer they go untreated. This book will take you through several types of heart disease, what you can do about preventing them, and how you can manage your condition through lifestyle changes.

What Is Heart Disease?

"Heart disease" (or cardiac disease) is a blanket term for the many ailments that the heart can have. These ailments include blockage, poor circadian rhythm, poor oxygenation, and other issues. Heart disease is deadly; it is the leading cause of death in the United States, the United Kingdom, Canada, and Australia. In the United States, nearly ¼ of all deaths are caused by heart disease.

Below are several types of heart diseases and their causes.

Angina pectoris is a condition in which a section of the heart's muscles does not get adequate oxygen. Angina is a condition that causes that under-oxygenated area of muscle to feel tight and uncomfortable. It is caused by coronary artery disease, which is a condition in which the arteries are narrowed due to plaque buildup.

Arrhythmia is a problem with the regular rhythm of the heart. The heart can either beat too quickly, too slowly, too early during development, or completely sporadically. Heart beats are controlled by electrical signals from the brain. Arrhythmia is caused when the heart's electrical signals from the brain are not functioning correctly.

When the heart beats too fast it is called tachycardia. If the heart beats slower than normal it is called bradycardia. A heart beating too early is considered a premature contraction, while fibrillation is an irregular heartbeat. Irregular heartbeats can be a normal occurrence. For instance, your pulse beats faster when you are agitated or excited and it beats slower when you are calm or asleep. Constant, throughout-the-day irregularities are not healthy, however, and should be addressed. If untreated, arrhythmia can lead to other complications—like heart strain—and be lethal.

Congenital heart disease is the term used for a birth defect of the heart. There are variations in congenital heart disease, but most of them involve the valves leading to the heart. Blood flowing out of the left side of the heart to the rest of the body is red and full of oxygen. Blood returning from the body and flowing into the right side of the heart is deoxygenated and blue. From there it is transported to the lungs to pick up more oxygen, and then back to the left side of the heart to be disseminated through the body again.

Each time the blood flows from a large blood vessel into or away from the heart, it passes through a heart valve. There can be several complications with these valves. First, the tricuspid valve, which is the valve that is between the two chambers that are on the right side of the heart, may not be able to open wide enough for adequate flow. Or it may be absent, which would allow backflow. Second, the pulmonary valve, which is the valve that is between the lungs and the heart, may also be unable to open wide enough for adequate flow, or it may be altogether absent. Third, the aortic valve, which is the valve that is between the heart and the blood vessel that carries oxygenated blood to the rest of the body, may be unable to open wide enough.

Septal defects, a congenital heart disease, are holes between the heart's two chambers. This passageway causes abnormal blood flow. Obstruction defects are when there is a blockage of normal blood flow. Cyanotic heart disease is a birth defect that results in low blood oxygen levels.

Coronary artery disease is when the arteries that bring blood and other things into the heart become damaged or diseased. These arteries supply the heart with oxygen, blood, and nutrients. They are most commonly affected by plaque deposits (which are build ups of cholesterol) that accumulate in the arteries and cause blockage, limiting the amount of oxygen the heart can receive. This is a precursor to heart attack, and has the same symptoms of chest pain and shortness of breath.

Dilated cardiomyopathy is a dilation of the heart chambers due to a weak heart muscle. When this happens, blood cannot be pumped through the heart regularly. This is most commonly caused because of a blockage in the main pumping chamber (the left ventricle), or coronary heart disease.

This condition can come without symptoms, but can be life threatening. It is a common cause of heart failure because the heart is unable to supply the body with enough blood to continue functioning. It can also cause arrhythmia and blood clots. This condition can affect anyone, even children and infants (http://www.mayoclinic.org/ diseases-conditions/dilated-cardiomyopathy/basics/definition/con-20032887).

Myocardial infarction is more commonly referred to as a heart attack, cardiac infarction, or coronary thrombosis. It occurs when one or both of the arteries that bring blood to the heart is blocked. The heart is starved of oxygenated blood and, if it does not get oxygen, that part of the heart dies. It can also be the result of a heart spasm or sudden narrowing of the artery. Myocardial infarction literally translates as "death of heart muscle."

Having a heart attack has been described as feeling like a large fist enclosing and tightening around the chest. It can be recognized by feeling short of breath, faint, dizzy, or nauseous (http://www.webmd.com/heart-disease/understanding-heart-attack-basics).

Congestive heart failure (in short, heart failure) is when the heart no longer has the ability to pump blood through the body. It usually affects one side of the body, but can sometimes affect both sides. High blood pressure or coronary artery disease can sometimes leave the heart too weak to pump blood strongly enough through the body, leading to heart failure.

Hypertrophic cardiomyopathy is caused by a thickening of the left ventricle, which makes it difficult for blood to leave the heart. Hypertrophic cardiomyopathy is a genetic disorder that has a 50% pass rate from mother/father to child. It is the leading cause of sudden death in athletes.

Mitral regurgitation (also called mitral valve regurgitation, mitral incompetence, and/or mitral insufficiency) is caused from blood flowing back into the heart because the mitral valve (a valve between the left atrium and left ventricle) does not close tightly enough. Patients often feel tired because blood is not flowing through the heart or body effectively. Mitral valve prolapse is when the mitral valve does not close, or expands upwards into the atrium. It is not considered life threatening, and does not require treatment unless it causes mitral regurgitation.

Pulmonary stenosis is caused from the pulmonary valve being too tight, making it difficult for blood to pump from the right ventricle into the pulmonary artery. Treatment is needed when the pressure in the right ventricle is too high. Babies can turn blue in severe cases, but children often do not show symptoms.

<u>Signs, Symptoms, and Risk Factors</u>

What are the signs of heart disease? How can you tell whether you or a loved one suffers from any of the above conditions? Who is at the most risk for developing these conditions?

There are some common signs of a heart problem. In general, they are chest pain, trouble breathing, pain, numbness, weakness in the extremities, and/or pain in the neck or other areas of the upper body. Each specific condition requires different treatment and should be diagnosed and treated by a doctor as soon as possible.

Coronary artery disease, congestive heart failure, and heart attacks share similar symptoms. The most common is chest pain or angina. Angina is characterized by pressure, heaviness, discomfort, or a painful feeling in your chest, shoulders, arms, neck, throat, or back. It is commonly mistaken for heartburn. Other symptoms of coronary heart disease are dizziness, a quickening or irregular heartbeat, sweating, and/or shortness of breath.

Symptoms of a heart attack can last longer than 30 minutes. Symptoms can start gradually and worsen over time. Symptoms can be pain in the arm or breastbone, indigestion, sweating, vomiting, shortness of breath, or irregular heartbeats. Diabetics, and sometimes others, may have a heart attack with no symptoms at all. Immediate treatment of a heart attack is necessary to prevent further damage to the heart.

Heart valve diseases have some slightly different symptoms. Shortness of breath can occur during normal activities or when lying down flat. Chest discomfort may start with activity or when in cold air. If valve disease leads to heart failure, symptoms can include the swelling of ankles, feet, or abdomen, or dramatic weight gain. Someone can have severe valve disease without showing any signs or symptoms, or vice versa.

Symptoms of heart failure are similar to those of heart valve disease in that showing symptoms does not necessarily relate to the severity of the problem. Symptoms are shortness of breath, coughing a white mucus, ankle swelling, dizziness, irregular heartbeat, nausea, and/or chest pain.

Congenital heart defects are characterized by shortness of breath (especially during exercise) and other symptoms of heart failure. In children, symptoms can be poor weight gain, lung infections, an inability to exercise, fast breathing, or lack of eating. If blood is not moving around the body or is under-oxygenated, toes and fingers may appear bluish because of the poor flow and lack of oxygen.

Heart muscle disease may have no symptoms and may not cause any problems. However, symptoms can include chest pain, heart failure symptoms, fainting, fatigue, and palpitations, and can occur at any age.

Risk Factors
Newsmaxhealth.com has a great online "test" at this link:

http://www.simplehearttest.com/heartsurvey.aspx/?dkt_nbr=pfys1r9b

You can use it to learn where you fall on their heart risk scale. It rates you on factors such as age, family history, lifestyle habits, height, weight, and others. Their goal is to educate users on their current risks and increase awareness of the possibility of developing heart disease.

Some risk factors of heart disease are controllable, while others are not. The more risk factors you have, the more likely you are to suffer from cardiovascular disease. Some risk factors put you at greater risk than others. Uncontrollable risk factors include the fact that men are more likely to have heart disease than women. Likewise, Caucasians are less likely to suffer from heart disease than any other race. Other uncontrollable factors are age, family history, and menopause (http://www.webmd.com/heart-disease/guide/heart-disease-symptoms).

But some controllable risk factors such as smoking, lack of physical exercise, obesity, stress and anger, poor cholesterol levels, and uncontrolled diabetes can greatly reduce your risk for heart disease if treated.

Making some lifestyle changes can dramatically reduce one's risk for heart disease and improve health. Smokers, for example, are two times more likely to suffer heart disease than non-smokers. Secondhand smoke is also a risk factor. Improving your cholesterol levels can reduce your chances of heart disease as well. A diet low in saturated or trans fats, cholesterol, and sugars will help, as will regular exercise.

Most people should exercise for 30 minutes each day. Along with exercise, eating foods low in sodium and high in antioxidants can lower your risk for heart disease. Fruits, vegetables, and whole grains can help you achieve a more heart-healthy diet (http://www.webmd.com/heart-disease/risk-factors-heart-disease).

The Connection with Diabetes

There are some terrible realities that patients with diabetes should know about. Damage to blood vessels from high blood pressure makes diabetic patients two times more likely to develop heart problems than people without diabetes. Diabetics tend to develop heart problems at a younger age, and two out of three die from heart disease or stroke.

Diabetics are especially susceptible to coronary artery disease caused by plaque buildup in the arteries. Sudden blockage by cholesterol plaque can cause a heart attack. Congestive heart failure is often caused by coronary artery disease, which is where the heart loses the ability to pump blood.

Additional risk factors are especially dangerous for diabetics. Metabolic syndrome is a name given to certain risk factors, namely high blood pressure, high blood sugar, poor cholesterol levels, high triglycerides, and belly fat (all of which increase the risk of heart disease). Often times all risk factors occur together, in that obesity leads to diabetics, who likely have high blood pressure.

Diabetic patients should also be aware of family member history concerning heart disease, as this will increase the risk even more—along with smoking and unhealthy diets.

In order to reduce the risk of heart disease, diabetics should follow the ABC's of diabetes treatment: A1c levels should be less than seven, blood pressure should be less than 130 over 80, and cholesterol should be less than 100 LDL and greater than 40 HDL.

Warning Signs (Stroke and Heart Attack)

What some may not realize is that a heart attack may not happen all at once, as is often depicted. In fact, many patients have heart attack symptoms and wait too long before seeking medical attention. It is important for people who have symptoms of a heart attack to seek medical attention quickly.

A study shows that 50% of people wait more than four hours from the first sign of symptoms before seeking medical attention. You should wait no more than five minutes, because if it is a sudden-onset heart attack, that is as much time as you have to avoid serious complications. Remember, it is never bad to be on the safe side, especially with something so serious (http://www.heart.org/HEARTORG/Conditions/911-Warnings-Signs-of-a-Heart-Attack_UCM_305346_SubHome Page.jsp).

Here are some common warnings signs of heart attacks:

Chest discomfort, or even pain, that starts at the center of the chest and lasts for more than just a few minutes. It can even go away and come back several times. This discomfort will feel like an unusual pressure, fullness, squeezing inside your chest, or simply pain.

Other upper body discomfort, such as that in the back, neck, jaw, stomach, or arms, can also indicate heart attack. While these pains can be caused by other things like working out or stress, be mindful that they can also indicate something more serious. Know your body and, when something is out of place, get help. Shortness of breath or pained breathing can also indicate heart attack, even without also feeling chest or other body pains. Other signs include feeling lightheaded or nauseous, and breaking out in a cold sweat (http://www.heart.org/HEARTORG/Conditions/911-Warnings-Signs-of-a-Heart-Attack_UCM_305346_SubHomePage.jsp).

Common signs of stroke are drooping of the face, weakness in the arms, and having difficulty speaking. If someone cannot smile with both sides of their face, raise their arms above their head (if they normally could), or speak normally, they may be suffering from a heart attack.

Some patients mistake heart attack symptoms for less serious ailments such as indigestion. If you feel you have symptoms of a heart attack, it is best to seek treatment. If you are experiencing symptoms of uncomfortable pressure or pain in the chest area at varying severity, shortness of breath, nausea, cold sweat, or pain in other areas of the upper body, you may be having a heart attack. Women may also experience fatigue, nausea, and dizziness.

Physically managing your heart health to prevent heart complications involves regular exercise or activity and eating a healthy diet. This two-pronged approach will keep you from building up unnecessary fat that puts pressure and strain on your organs (including your heart), and it will keep strengthening your heart. Just like any other muscle, the heart needs to be exercised to stay in good shape.

Eating healthy is also a necessary part of heart health. A diet that is mindful of your heart health can reduce your susceptibility to stroke or heart attack by up to 80%. The key is to manage weight gain, blood sugar levels, cholesterol, and blood pressure to keep unnecessary strain off of the heart (http://www.helpguide.org/life/healthy_ diet_heart_disease_stroke.htm.)

Health Diet Substitutions
Eating whole grains, low fat dairy, fruits, vegetables, lean meats, fish, nuts and beans, and avoiding red meats in your diet will improve heart health. Staying away from high-calorie yet low nutrient foods will prevent unnecessary weight gain, which is a considerable contributing factor to heart complications. You should also limit your intake of foods that are high in sodium, trans fats, and saturated fats, as these raise your cholesterol.

Eating foods that contain a lot of sodium will raise your blood pressure. Continual elevated blood pressure is known as hypertension, which is a serious heart issue. It is a leading cause of strokes, heart attacks, and heart failure. Too much sodium intake leads to other complications, such as osteoporosis, obesity, kidney disease, kidney stones, cancer, and water retention. It can worsen the symptoms of asthma and diabetes (http://www.actiononsalt.org.uk/less/Health/).

Changing bad habits in your diet may not be easy, but it is necessary if you want to avoid heart trouble in the future. A lot of weak spots in our diets can be replaced with healthier alternatives. Instead of eating red meats that are high in fat, eat lean poultry and/or fish without cooking them in saturated or trans-fat oils. Avoid "deep fried" foods and opt for something that is either baked or grilled.

Chicken and turkey are both great sources of protein, but they contain much less fat than pork or hamburger meat. Eating fish three times a week is recommended for those with heart trouble because of the "good" (omega-3) fat it contains. Salmon and tuna are considered a good source of nutrients that promote heart health. You can exchange your whole milk (which is high in sugar and fat) for low fat 1% milk or soy milk.

If you are in the mood for something sweet, consider health snack alternatives. Instead of having a bag of chips or a candy bar as a snack, consider eating a handful of berries over a small bowl of yogurt. The berries and yogurt will make you feel fuller longer, and they are void of the fat that is in processed snacks. If you are in the mood for something chocolaty, eat dark chocolate instead of milk or white chocolate. Chocolates that are 70% cocoa help improve your heart health and satisfy those with a sweet tooth.

It is also believed that a glass of red wine will improve cardiovascular health because of its antioxidants. But, any alcohol in excess will have adverse effects on the body.

What role does water play?

Drinking water helps to ensure that your body is well hydrated. This is especially important if you plan to do the recommended 30 minutes of exercise per day. At the baseline, you should be consuming at least eight cups of water every day (http://www. mayoclinic.org/healthy-living/nutrition-and-healthy-eating/in-depth/water/art-20044256?pg=2), but water intake needs vary by person based on factors such as health, gender, weight, and others. A formula method for determining your water needs based on weight is to take your weight in pounds, divide it in half, and drink that many OUNCES of water per day.

For example, Susie weighs 150 pounds. Susie would divide her weight in half, which would be 75 pounds. She would need to drink at least 75 OUNCES of water each day. Since a cup is about eight ounces, Susie would need to drink almost nine cups of water every day.

But exercise increases your need for water. For every 30 minutes of exercise, you should drink another 1.5–2.5 cups. Here's another example: Tim weighs 200 pounds and started working out for 30 minutes a day. His base need for water is 100 OUNCES (200 pounds divided by 2). This would be about 13 glasses of water a day. With his exercise, he needs 2.5 more glasses of water, so overall he should be drink 15 to 15.5 glasses of water each day.

<u>Where Should I Start?</u>

Calorie counting is a good way to jump-start your heart-healthy diet. But keep in mind that calorie counting must be accompanied by good nutrition. We might all agree that only eating one cheeseburger a day will reduce your calorie intake, but it will not be healthy for you, for a few reasons. First, not all calories are "created equal." Some foods are much better at making you feel satisfied or jump-starting your metabolism. Other calories, like those from sugary, processed, or high-sodium foods, are not. Even if it is the same number of calories, it does not have the same health effects.

Second, "starving" yourself is not the way to lose weight. If your body feels like you are not getting enough calories, it will store up reserves of fat and sugar because it feels like it is in an emergency situation. Eating healthy does not mean being hungry. Eating healthy means replacing less nutritious foods in your diet with more nutritious options. Simply eating better will improve even the worst diets.

A sample of a good, heart-healthy day might be to try, for breakfast, mixing common breakfast foods with blueberries (such as pancakes, waffles, or oatmeal). Mix spinach with a combination of nuts and other greens for a healthy mid-day lunch. And bake salmon in the oven for dinner along with healthy sides like cooked carrots and brown rice.

Eating healthy is a big part of keeping your heart healthy, but it should be combined with regular cardiovascular exercise. Riding a bike, kayaking, swimming, using an elliptical machine, running, or brisk walking are all forms of aerobic exercise that will improve your heart's function. Doctors recommend 30 minutes a day of increased activity to help your heart stay in shape. Losing excess body fat, especially around the midsection, can dramatically decrease your risk level for heart disease and diabetes. Combining exercise and healthy eating is a sure way to improve heart health.

Steps to Reducing High Blood Pressure and Unclogging Your Arteries

High blood pressure is defined as a reading of at least 140/90 mmHg. Anything higher than this can put you at risk for several health conditions, including heart disease and stroke. Blood pressure can be controlled with lifestyle changes and/or medicine prescribed by your doctor. Lowering your blood pressure can reduce your risk of developing or worsening a heart condition.

According to the Mayo Clinic, it may be as simple as losing 10 pounds to start keeping your blood pressure in check. This is a small goal that should just be the start of your lifestyle changes. If you have the weight to lose, then the more weight you lose, the lower your blood pressure will go. If you are overweight or obese, losing weight may also make any blood pressure medicine you are taking more effective.

You can start losing weight with mild exercise and a healthy diet.

Talk to your doctor about where you are and what your realistic goals should be. They can help you determine these things, taking into account your body mass index, your medications, and your expectations. You can talk to your doctor about what foods will work best for you (because some can interfere with medicines) and what kind of recommendations they have for exercise. In general, doctors recommend about 30 minutes of mild to moderate exercise per day. That may be as easy as taking a brisk walk up and down the street and doing chores around your house.

Another tip is to lessen your sodium intake. Reducing just a small amount of salt in your diet can reduce your blood pressure by about 8 mmHg. Processed, preserved foods and restaurant foods usually have the highest amounts of sodium. Try to keep your sodium intake to less than 2,300 mg per day. As you get older, your salt intake should decrease. By age 50, you should be taking in less than 1,500 mg per day.

Lowered blood pressure can also be attributed to lowered stress levels. Moments of stress increase your blood pressure for a short amount of time. Being overweight puts you at increased risk for high blood pressure, because your heart has to work harder to pump blood throughout your body. Because of that, you should be extra careful to keep your stress down so that your blood pressure does not rise unnecessarily.

Stress can be kept at bay in several different ways. The first would be to eat a healthy diet. Eating well will make you feel fuller, more energized, and—quite literally—happier. Exercise will also make you feel more relaxed. There are also other ways to control stress, like deep breathing exercises and meditation.

Another factor that could be causing you stress is lack of adequate sleep. It is important for adults to get between seven and a half to nine hours of sleep each night. Getting less than that can make you groggy, lethargic, cranky, or dysfunctional. All of these factors lead to increased agitation and stress.

Several things can disrupt sleep, such as overworking yourself, going to bed at irregular times, or snoring during your sleep. To help with a sleeping problem, try a few simple steps.

First, get used to going to bed early, so that you can get enough sleep before getting up to start the next day. Remember, seven and a half to nine hours is the magic range. Second, sleep in a space that is free of disturbance. Keep your phone away from you at night so that you do not stay up checking emails or playing games. Third, try and go to sleep and wake up at the same time every day. Having a regular schedule will keep your body on track to actually fall asleep when you want to, instead of lying awake in bed for hours.

If none of these measures work and you are constantly tired during the day, try asking a family member or sleeping partner whether they notice you snoring or waking up frequently during the night. There are several ways you can control moderate snoring. If it is not something you can control on your own, you may want to see a sleep doctor about your problem. They may discover that you have sleep apnea, a condition in which you wake up several times during the night because your airways are blocked when lying down.

You should also decrease your intake of alcohol, caffeine, and smoking. Your doctor can work with you on which of these factors will affect you most. Together, you can work up a blood pressure reduction plan.

There are also some nutrients that may help lower high blood pressure.

Potassium, calcium, magnesium, fish oils, and garlic all help some people to lower their blood pressure. There are many fruits, vegetables, fish, and dairy foods that have enough potassium that you can get your needed amounts from diet alone. Unlike some other necessary nutrients, it probably is not necessary to take potassium supplements. In cultures where calcium is rarely eaten, the population generally has higher blood pressure. Calcium can be found in yogurt, low fat milk, and cheeses.

Magnesium is present is leafy green vegetables, whole grains, nuts, seeds, and dry peas and beans. The required amounts are usually found in a typical healthy diet, so, just as with potassium, supplements should not be necessary.

Remember that it is always important to talk to your doctor before making any major diet changes. Your diet can greatly affect your body and any medications you are taking, so you need to know if you could possibly have any adverse reactions. Dietary supplements are the same. Having too much potassium, magnesium, or any other nutrient can be bad for you. To avoid overdoses of these nutrients, talk to your doctor to determine what you are already getting and if you need any more.

Superfoods—Eat Your Way to a Healthy Heart

It is important to understand that no one single food is going to give you a healthy heart. The idea is to improve your overall diet, while eliminating certain unhealthy foods. We've chosen seven of the best foods for a heart-healthy diet, and we are going to explain their effects on the body and why they deserve to be on this elite list.

Remember, before making any major lifestyle or diet changes, consult your doctor or dietician. They should know how the different foods you are eating will affect you or any medication that you are taking.

Fatty fish like salmon, sardines, herring, lake trout, albacore tuna, and mackerel contain a lot of omega-3 fatty acids, which are great for your heart health. These fish can lower the risk of irregular heartbeats (arrhythmia), plaque buildup and obstruction in the arteries (atherosclerosis), and also decreases triglycerides. You should eat fatty fish at least two times per week, per the American Heart Association's recommendation.

People who have coronary artery disease or high triglycerides may not be getting enough fatty acids through diet alone. For you, the American Heart Association suggests taking supplements. Outside of fish, you can find omega-3 fatty acids in dietary supplement form.

Oatmeal is a great addition to your diet for many reasons. Even though it is high in carbohydrates, it has a low glycemic index rating. The glycemic index rates foods on a scale of 1 to 100. The traditional "simple carbs" rate high on the list, with greater than 55 points. The higher on the list you go, the faster the body can turn that food into sugar and absorb it into the blood, hence raising the blood sugar level. It is preferable if it takes the body a while to convert the carbs into sugar before absorbing them. Traditional "complex carbs" have lower ratings under 55 points and take longer to absorb. Oatmeal is one of the foods that ranks low on the index.

Oatmeal is also high in soluble fiber. Soluble fiber is very healthy because it absorbs cholesterol that is in the bloodstream before it can be absorbed, thereby lowering cholesterol. Other whole grains, even though they have carbs, can be good for you as long as they contain the whole grain. Having the grain intact makes it harder for the body to dissolve and absorb as sugar. Oatmeal that is sweetened with sugar, or instant oatmeal, should be avoided in favor of "old-fashioned" or "quick-cooking" oats.

Berries such as blueberries, strawberries, raspberries, blackberries, and acai berries can lead to a lower risk of heart complications. In a recent study done by the Harvard School of Public Health (HSPH) and the University of East Anglia, researchers found that women who eat at least three servings of strawberries and/or blueberries are at lower risk of having heart attacks. Heart attack is the leading cause of death for women, and women are more susceptible to heart attack than men.

Berries contain antioxidants and polyphenols, and are a good source of soluble fiber. All of these combine to help the body fight chronic diseases, like heart disease and cancer.

Research followed the eating habits of 93,600 female nurses aged 25–42 years. These nurse's eating habits were followed for 18 years, while researchers checked in on them every four years. The original study can be found at http://circ.ahajournals.org/content/127/2/188.full. Those who ate three servings of berries per week were less likely to develop heart complications.

Citrus fruits, such as oranges and grapefruits, are known to lower the risk of heart disease due to their high vitamin C content. Vitamin C is a great source of folate and potassium. Potassium strengthens muscles (the heart is a muscle!) and folate promotes red blood cell production.

The flavonoids in citrus fruits also have antioxidants that are known to neutralize free radicals in a way that protects the heart against disease. Citrus flavonoids can improve blood flow through the coronary arteries, inhibit blood clots from forming in the arteries (which would impede blood flow), and prevent the oxidation of bad cholesterol, known as LDL. Lowering bad cholesterol is a great quality because forming cholesterol is one of the first steps in building up plaque in the arteries.

Polyunsaturated fats can help reduce "bad" cholesterol (LDL), and that can reduce your risk of heart attack and/or stroke. It also provides the necessary fats and omega-3 and omega-6 acids that your body cannot produce by itself. Poly- and mono-unsaturated fats are much better for you than saturated and trans fats, because those fats can raise your cholesterol.

Nuts, including walnuts, almonds, peanuts, macadamia nuts, and pistachios, all contain fiber, which is good for your heart. Walnuts even have a high content of omega-3 fatty acids. Nuts may be viewed negatively because they have a lot of fat, but they have been linked to reducing body fat, which in turn promotes heart health. Be sure that you are consuming nuts that do not have a lot of added sugar.

Legumes like beans, lentils, and peas are good sources of protein that are low in fat. In a 2001 study reported by the US National Library of Medicine and the National Institute of Health, eating legumes four or more times per week was linked to a 22% lower chance of developing coronary heart disease than only eating legumes once per week. It was also linked to an 11% decrease in the risk of developing cardiovascular disease.

The study followed 9,362 men and women over 19 years. These participants were free of heart disease and cardiovascular disease at the start of the study. It is thought that perhaps the copper found in legumes contributes to this health benefit.

In another study published by the same institution, legumes were researched for their effects on blood sugar levels. A total of 121 participants who had type II diabetes (the type that usually forms later in life due to poor diet, high blood sugar, and excess fat) were sorted into two groups. The first group increased their consumption of legumes by one cup per day. The second group was to increase their insoluble fiber consumption in the form of whole-wheat products.

This study lasted for three months and measured the hemoglobin A1c values in the patients, as well as their coronary heart disease risk. While both diets decreased the hemoglobin A1C levels (a good outcome), the legume diet decreased them by 0.2% more than the whole-wheat diet. The legume diet also lowered systolic blood pressure more effectively than the whole-wheat diet. The study concluded that a diet high in legumes versus a diet that is high in "good" carbs was a better way to lower hemoglobin A1c levels and to reduce the risk of cardiovascular disease.

Reversing Heart Disease for Life

Heart disease causes actual physical damage to the heart and surrounding blood vessels. So, the question is, can that damage be reversed? Can it be slowed down or stopped?

The answer is yes and no. It is unlikely, after several years or decades of progress towards heart disease, that you will be able to erase its effects completely. It is possible, however, to slow down, halt, and reverse some of the effects. The quicker the heart disease is identified and treated, the easier it will be to "cure."

Doctor Dean Ornish (Dr. Oz), president and founder of the Preventive Medicine Research Institute, has written several books, one of which details his plan to reverse heart disease.

His book, *The Spectrum*, chronicles the lives of heart disease patients who were on the list to undergo heart transplants. They had the worst possible conditions and were at the last possible step they could take. While in that position, they started Doctor Ornish's program.

He reports that it only took a month for the patients' hearts to start pumping normally and for blood flow to improve. He attributes that success to significant lifestyle changes. Artery blockage lessened and patients continued to improve, even five years after the start of the program.

Doctor Ornish's program consists of walking at least half an hour a day, or for one full hour three times a week. He also incorporates yoga and meditation to improve blood flow and reduce stress. He places a heavy emphasis on eating healthy. His program divides foods into five categories, from most to least healthy.

To be most healthy, the doctor says that you would become a vegetarian. You would replace your meats with fruits, vegetables, whole grains, nonfat dairy, egg whites, legumes, nuts, and possibly soy. It is important to avoid sugars, fats, and processed carbohydrates. The point is to eat natural foods is their natural forms, and avoid preservatives, added sugars, or excess fat as much as you possibly can.

Doctor Ornish says that success with his program requires dedication and motivation. Diet and lifestyle changes are not easy, but the health benefits can be invaluable. Others suggest that being too strict with your new lifestyle and expectations can prove to be disappointing should you at some point waver from them. The goal is to make improvement and stick to realistic expectations. Getting discouraged and giving up completely will land you right back where you were to begin with, or even worse off.

Alternative Treatments for Heart Disease

If you are looking for an alternative to taking a pill for a heart condition, some recent studies and research believe they have found other ways of managing or preventing heart disease. A lot of alternative treatment deals with managing your stress levels. In our high-paced world, stress is inevitable; however, being able to find a sense of calm can help you better control a heart condition and promote longevity for the most important organ in your body. In addition to managing your stress, acupuncture treatment has had significant success in reducing the effects of some heart conditions. There are always treatment options available, and a cardiologist can certainly put you on the right track to managing a heart condition.

Acupuncture treatment has been around since 6000 BCE. Its methods and legitimacy in the Western world have improved a lot since its origin in imperial China. Acupuncture is a treatment that involves puncturing the skin with tiny needles in certain areas of the body to alleviate pain or other conditions. Researchers now know that acupuncture treatment can be used to stimulate nerve endings affecting the brain to do something useful for the person receiving the treatment. It has been used on headaches, back pain, nausea, and dental patients to cure ailments.

Electroacupuncture, the use of battery operated needles for acupuncture, can now be used to lower blood pressure with weekly tests. Electroacupunture is being used around patients' elbows and knee areas at different frequencies and pressures to affect the response of the brain's cardiovascular areas. Research shows that the practice has managed to drop patients' blood pressure by 20 points.

This compares favorably to the use of traditional medicines, with very little in the way of side effects. It is not possible to completely rid someone of hypertension, so acupuncture treatment must be done weekly in order to keep blood pressure patients' levels down. More blood pressure patients may soon be turning to this type of treatment to help reduce the amount of medications they have to take— helping the kidneys and reducing side effects that are often just as cumbersome as the condition itself.

Most people are aware that stress is a mental illness, but what they may not know is how much that stress is actually affecting their physical health as well. Stress from daily problems can literally cause a heart attack. The brain and its ability to handle the outside world can cause more physical damage than mental. Managing this stress is hard, but can be aided with medication.

With practice, it can also be treated without medication. Studies by the Institute of HeartMath showed that learning stress reduction methods can lower someone's blood pressure almost completely. In one test subject, their high blood pressure was completely eliminated. Most subjects saw a decrease of 12%.

When you are stressed, your body releases hormones such as adrenaline and cortisol, which cause damage to your heart over time. On the other hand, when your stress levels are managed, the body releases or creates more heart-healthy hormones, which keep the heart running normally. Of course, the other hormones are important for certain situations where your body needs to react quickly in high stress situations. But too much (from a lack of control) will lead to heart problems.

In an effort to manage stress, there is an easy method to learn called "positive refocusing" in which you can reverse what type of hormones your body uses in stressful situations. When you begin to feel stressed or anxious, take a moment to relax and meditate on the thought or problem that is stressful. Take some deep breaths for a few minutes while focusing on slowing down your heart rate. Afterwards, think on some happy thoughts—a fun time you had with someone you love or care about, a favorite hobby, event, or accomplishment. This may be hard to do the first few times you try it, but over time it will become quicker and easier. You will certainly notice a difference in your stress levels, as well as your blood pressure.

Patients in the study were able to reduce the amount of blood pressure medication they took, and in turn were able to reduce stress and the added side effects of their medications. Using this method is highly beneficial and worth a try— no prescription needed.

Tai chi is another old Chinese method of martial arts that uses smooth motions at a constant speed. This method uses a variety of postures that flow smoothly in a slow, focused, and fluent motion. It is a low-impact and self-paced exercise that can be done by people of any physical skill level or age. It is very good on joints, and is even good for those with arthritis or other physical ailments preventing them from doing more common workouts.

Tai chi has been known to have many positive effects on the body. It can reduce stress, increase energy, strengthen muscles, improve muscle definition, and improve pulmonary function. It has been known to improve sleep, the immune system, and joint pain. It can also lower LDL cholesterol and blood pressure, and heighten the overall well being of the practitioner.

Tai chi can be done in many different ways and in many different venues. You can buy DVDs and do it at home, take classes in local health or community centers, or purchase books. It is something that can be performed outdoors, in short amounts, or for long periods of time. Tai chi can focus on the martial arts or just on improving health, so pick the method you are most interested in. This stress-relieving exercise is a very diverse form of exercise and can be used by anyone to help improve not only your heart health, but many other areas of your physical and mental health as well (http://www.mayoclinic.org/healthy-living/stress-management/in-depth/tai-chi/ art-20045184) (http://www.prevention.com/health/health-concerns/heart-health-best-alternative-therapies).

In the end, many alternative treatments for heart disease come down to managing stress, diet, and exercise. Being able to drop weight, eat foods that promote heart health, and control hormones in your body will decrease your risk for heart disease or slow down ailments that eventually lead to heart problems like high blood pressure.

Heart Disease Wrap-up

     The first step towards combating heart disease is to be diagnosed by your doctor. It is important to know exactly what your condition is and the best way to fight it. Several steps can be taken, including taking the right medications, changing your diet, or changing your lifestyle.

     Here are a few tips that were described in this book:

     Eat a diet that is low in fat and sodium. Fat increases cholesterol and sodium increases blood pressure. Cholesterol can build up in your arteries in the form of plaque and cause blockages to your heart. Instead, replace these foods with healthy substitutions like lean meats, fish, fruit, leafy green vegetables, "good" carbs, nuts, and beans.

     Exercise at least 30 minutes per day. In today's age, when we do not have to walk or bike from place to place or work to procure our food, we are living a much more sedentary lifestyle than anyone in the past. To make up for this, we need to actively exercise more. This can be as simple as doing half an hour of yoga or taking a brisk walk. Any little bit will help—even getting up to do chores around your home, or walking out and checking the mail every day.

     Lower your stress as much as possible. There are so many things in our daily lives that can stress us out. There's work, school, friends, family, bills, etc. We need to find healthy ways to channel that stress away from us. At the same time, we need to make sure that we are getting enough sleep every night. Adults are recommended to have between seven and a half and nine hours each night. Getting enough good sleep ensures that you are rested, alert, and at your physical peak.

Printed in Great Britain
by Amazon